The Nordic Method

A workout system for community-based, functional strength training

ALF BERLE

ISBN-10: 1535535199
ISBN-13: 978-1535535199

Rimfjord AS | Nordic Method
Bergen, Norway
www.nordicmethod.com

DEDICATION

To my old track coach, Ingvald Ytrehus: Thank you for your decades of outstanding effort; your patience, diligence, enthusiasm and creative training methods. I am forever in your debt, as are many.

To the H.O.T.CH.I.C.K.S. of Palo Alto, CA, and the Canadian superwomen Lindsey Hoole and Susan Leech in particular: Thank you for your friendship, support, and inexplicable tolerance for pervasive Nordic grumpiness. Without you there would be no training manual.
Keep grinding the Viking battle-axe!

DISCLAIMER

Repeat after me:
I hereby declare that by embarking on the training program described in this book,
I assume full responsibility for my own health and wellbeing.
I will make a consistent effort and work hard to improve my fitness.
I will use this program with care and common sense and listen to what my body is telling me.
I will blame no one but myself if I fail to do so.
I will congratulate myself on my successes and help others succeed to the best of my ability.

CONTENTS

ACKNOWLEDGMENTS

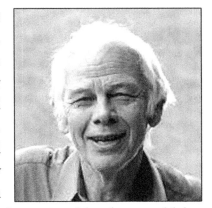

The most important source of inspiration for the Nordic Method is one man: My track coach through my teenage years, Ingvald Ytrehus. Growing up in a tiny town way out in the hicks in Norway, the choice of sports was pretty limited. Soccer was the main thing. Few opted for the more strenuous track training. Still the team consistently performed extremely well on national level, thanks to the quiet genius of Ingvald. His methods were a curious mix of traditional and innovative, based primarily on his vast experience; he was never one for being overly academic with his ideas. Gymnastic moves, bodyweight strength training, sprinting, jumping, throwing, basic Olympic weightlifting, and occasional hard manual labor (!) were all part of the training. Ingvald always participated, only standing on the sidelines when a critical examination was required. He continues to live as he taught: Not so long ago I spotted him coming out of the woods carrying a sizeable tree trunk, probably close to 200 pounds. At the age of 75, after invasive hip surgery, he was still strong and vigorous, with muscles that appeared forged from steel wire. He has thoroughly earned my gratitude and respect, and his influence runs deep.

Regarding some of the specific workout programs, a source of inspiration has been Mark Twight's *The Spartan Warrior Workout*, penned and adapted by Dave Randolph and published by Ulysses Press. Some of the workouts in the second half of the book are inspired by *The Spartan Warrior Workout*. It's a remarkably good program for general strength conditioning, as can be witnessed from the outstanding physical shape of the actors in the movie *The 300*, but it does require access to quite a bit of equipment.

Some of the kettlebell stuff owes its legacy to Pavel Tsatsouline's *Russian Kettlebell Challenge (RKC)* and several derivatives thereof. A former instructor for Soviet Union Special Forces, Pavel is considered the primary advocate for bringing modern-day kettlebell training to the U.S. Additional inspiration has also been found aplenty in Paul Wade's *Convict Conditioning 1 & 2*; *C-Mass*; and in several books by the Kavadlo brothers Al and Danny. All of these books are published by Dragon Door and are highly recommended as outstanding references for kettlebell and bodyweight strength training.

For general fitness/ strength conditioning, no major fitness trend has in my opinion hit the mark better than CrossFit. It is perhaps not perfect, among other things diving too deeply into the high-intensity/ high-load training segment for my taste, but it can be very good indeed with the right instructors. I like it. It works. CrossFit has managed to create a sticky and lasting fitness culture based on great fundamental principles. I have however largely refrained from adopting the practice of giving female names to particularly grueling workouts or tests, although I'll admit to finding CrossFit founder Greg Glassman's explanation of this quite intriguing: "Any workout that leaves you out of breath, flat on your back, staring up at the sky and wondering what the heck happened, deserves a woman's name".

1. INTRODUCTION

We all know what fitness is, right? "Sure, fitness is… well, it's… ya'know. Being in great shape. Being fit." Indeed. It is not so straightforward, apparently. Looking the word up in a dictionary will provide a definition along the lines of:

fitness <noun>

1. health.

2. capability of the body of distributing inhaled oxygen to muscle tissue during increased physical effort.

3. also called Darwinian fitness. *Biology*

   a. the genetic contribution of an individual to the next generation's gene pool relative to the average for the population, usually measured by the number of offspring or close kin that survive to reproductive age.

   b. the ability of a population to maintain or increase its numbers in succeeding generations.

Now, the latter definition can probably be dismissed for our purpose, unless you have a very detached perspective on what life is all about. As for the first one: Is fitness and health necessarily the same? It is probably possible for a healthy person to not be particularly fit, at least as I understand the terms. And it is certainly possible for a person with a severe illness, e.g. cancer, to have a very high level of fitness without being healthy. My friend Jon, 65 years at the time, outran me up a mountainside while he was undergoing a period of heavy chemotherapy. He wasn't healthy at all, but damn sure fit.

The second definition equates fitness to cardiovascular capacity. This is valid to some extent, but also excludes many top performing athletes. People who compete in sports that require considerable strength and power rely more on the ability of the muscles to perform in an anaerobic state, i.e. not using oxygen. Although many will certainly have a very decent 'capability to distribute inhaled oxygen', it is secondary. What about an Olympic sprinter or a world-class powerlifter? Are these people not fit?

In the year 2000, coach Greg Glassman founded the CrossFit movement from his renegade gym in Santa Cruz, CA. The problem of defining fitness was recognized from the beginning: "Perhaps the definition of fitness doesn't include strength, speed, power, and coordination though that seems rather odd", writes Glassman. He moves on to define fitness as our competency in ten recognized general physical skills: Cardiovascular/respiratory endurance, speed, stamina, strength, flexibility, power, coordination, agility, balance, and accuracy. I believe this definition originated from the gentlemen Crawley and Evans of exercise machine producer Dynamax, although it is of no great consequence. The definition is still a good one. Glassman's point of view is nicely summarized in his article 'What is fitness?', published in the CrossFit Journal of October 2002. It is well worth a read.

There is a small issue here though, as pointed out by one of my favorite authors on this subject, the highly educated gentleman and coach extraordinaire, Dan John: The CrossFit definition still doesn't quite capture the fact that, say, a discus thrower can be fit despite lacking significant cardiovascular endurance or stamina. John uses a definition by Dr. Phil Maffetone that fitness is *the ability to do a particular task*, which would encompass high-level athletes in any field.

I'll venture into unchartered territory and combine these two definitions. We then arrive at:

1. Specific physical fitness:

   The ability to perform a particular task by mastering necessary physical skills.

2. General physical fitness:

   Competency in all of the ten physical skills; cardiovascular/respiratory endurance; speed; stamina; strength; flexibility; power; coordination; agility; balance; and accuracy.

For most of us who are simply trying to stay 'in shape', looking toward the definition of general physical fitness seems most appropriate. For instance, I no longer dream of being an Olympic sprinter (supreme speed and power) or a champion dart player (supreme accuracy), but I do dream of continuing to keep up with my kids in the playground without becoming injured, bedridden or dead, and I would like to be able to carry a heavy backpack in rough terrain at the age of 80. A functional level of general fitness it is, then, and preferably by means that are sustainable for decades.

Forty, Fat and Finished?

The journey into fitness – or out of it, for that matter – is a personal one. As individuals, we work out for a variety of different reasons. Common motivations include weight loss or fat loss, the promise of longevity, or a desire to avoid the aches and pains that often result from inactivity. A purpose statement that you'll often hear is "I just want to tone up a little", an indirect way of saying "I want to look good naked". This one is pretty universal. Life in modern society doesn't necessarily make it easy for us, though. A lot of jobs require extended periods sitting still, and those that don't tend to have very monotonous motion patterns or involve unfavorable static positions. In many cities you can hardly get around without driving, and to relax we slump onto the couch and turn on the TV. It's a quagmire. Changing the situation requires decisive action.

Believe me, I've been there. For me, the turning point occurred on a beautiful summer day in 2008. My wife and I had invited some friends over for a meal and a few drinks. The beer was in the cooler and the barbecue was heating up. Then two of our friends arrived on bikes - they are a handsome couple a few years younger than me - he with his shirt off in the summer heat. My wife looked at him in awe and murmured, "Oh my, he's got a six-pack!" Realizing the Freudian slip, she glanced at me with a sheepish, yet not too apologetic grin on her face. That's when it struck me: I was fat. Not seriously overweight, just generally out of shape with a bit of everyday flab. I had no idea how it had happened: Up until that point I'd been a strapping and fit 20-year-old athlete, at least in my own mind. Now I woke up with a start and found that I was in my thirties, fat, and very nearly finished. It was the final drop. I had to get back in shape.

Vanity aside: There were a few rather more serious reasons as well. I was hurting, the kind of dull, persistent ache that a lot of office workers suffer from. It tends to start in the lower back or in the shoulder and neck area. For me it was behind the left shoulder blade, a hard knot that had been bothering me with increasing intensity for a couple of years. Chronic pain is very tiring, and will leave you exhausted and irritable, often resulting in additional painful conditions. It is a downward spiral. I'd tried anti-inflammatory medication, physical therapy, and chiropractic treatments. Nothing really worked for more than a few days. In the end I went to the chiropractor every other week and took drugs nearly every day to be able to sleep. Obviously, the treatment dealt with the symptoms rather than the cause. Activities that I used to enjoy tremendously, such as hiking, hunting and winter sports, were becoming increasingly challenging. In addition I tended to get injured every time I tried to do any sort of rigorous physical activity: Torn muscles, aching joints, tendonitis, plantar fasciitis... you name it. I was in my early thirties and worn down. Worst of all, I could not really blame it on age, although it certainly was tempting.

Back in college I was a track athlete. Admittedly not a particularly successful one, my best result being a single bronze medal in the national championships. But I trained hard as hell, perhaps too hard, eight or nine sessions a week for a total of 20 hours. I used to be able to squat more than 450 pounds (200kg) and do a 10.5 feet (3.2m) standing broad jump, and I could easily carry an 80-pound backpack for hours in rough terrain. I attended courses and seminars and got certified in general fitness coaching and track coaching, leading classes several times a week. I read up on sports nutrition and practiced a healthy dietary regime. Then suddenly my college days were over and reality set in. With no more competitions to work towards, my exercise regime gradually dwindled. There was nothing radical about the transition from fit to fattish. It happened the way it happens to most people: Graduated from college, got a job, found a girlfriend, had a kid, got married, got promoted, had more kids, got promoted again, and all of a sudden I'd been sitting firmly on my ass and hardly moving for the best part of 10 years. Add in a liberal serving of work-related and domestic stress and you have a recipe for disaster.

So what to do? Succumb to depression and just led it slide? No way! Go on a diet? Maybe, but I knew enough about nutrition and training to realize that this would only partially address the problem and probably not be a lasting solution. Instead, I turned to my experience in athletics and coaching and devised a plan. It would need to take into account the limited time available to a parent and working professional, and it would need to be sustainable for decades. Long term goals: No more stress-related pain; replace fat with muscle; be fit to do physical labor or non-extreme sports without the risk of injury; keep it up for half a century.

A succession of trials and errors ensued, as I researched and tested a number of training methods and exercise styles. Eventually, a system emerged that felt right for me. To compare it to known entities, it ended up as a hybrid with elements from Russian kettlebell training, track training, CrossFit, P90X and some archaic methods out of the Norwegian fjords. Now, several years later, I can truly say that it has worked - so far, at least. I am in great shape, in some ways better than I was as a competitive athlete. There are still issues to address, but I'm working on those and improving.

I'll freely admit this, though: The Nordic Method will make you a jack of all trades and master of none. You will not become brutally strong in absolute strength terms, but you will become stronger than most. You will not develop astonishing endurance, but you'll have the resources to deal with anything from moving furniture to a multi-day backpacking hike without issues. You will not become a trapeze artist, but your balance will improve and could help you avoid a broken hip sometime in the future. All in all you'll become quite good in quite a lot of different physical aspects. Frankly, I believe that this is what serves us best in the long term. Becoming very good at something very specific requires a high degree of specialization at the expense of other abilities that would be useful in everyday life. The Nordic Method on the other hand provides general fitness, and it's a model that will work for most people of average health and capability.

This book is dedicated to sharing the experiences I've made in the process of getting back into functional fitness, in the hope that it may inspire and help others. Will it work for everyone? Not necessarily, but it may provide guidance. It is not about building huge muscles. It is not about being the strongest person in the world or running ultra-marathons. It is about living life fully with a body that works.

2. THE NORDIC METHOD

Just before WW2, two brothers hiked into the mountains of Norway to cut peat. Times were hard and the supply of firewood was limited, hence the ancient practice of heating homes with dried peat was still in use. It was a nice, warm spring day, and the young men quickly went to work. After hours of hard labor, an accident happened: One of the men cut into his foot with the sharp peat shovel, leaving a deep, bleeding gash. There was no way he could walk, and they were a long way from the nearest farm. After dressing the wound as best they could, the younger of the two hoisted his brother up across his shoulders and carried him back home. 200 pounds additional weight, for 2 hours on rough trails: Feel free to try it!

The younger brother was my grandfather. He was impressively strong well into his seventies, whereupon he decided that he was now retired, sat down in a chair, and dwindled away. That particular generation, and many before them, had a considerable capacity for physical work, forged from a lifetime of manual labor. I distinctly remember my cousin's granddad, then in his late sixties, doing one-arm pull-ups with only the middle finger of his right hand hooked around a 5-inch nail. If you don't realize the raw power behind something like that, I recommend going into a gym and asking the most muscular guy there to do one. I think you'll have an epiphany.

These old-timers were true Vikings. Not huge and muscle-bound, mostly, but lean and hard as steel. The Nordic Method is a system built around functional strength and strength endurance training methods that have their roots in the Nordic way of life, from the Vikings to the modern-day society. In fairness though, the ancients never needed to train quite the way we do. Their physical foundation was secured through manual labor from a young age, on the farm and at sea, and by traversing the rugged terrains of Scandinavia. Hence, their actual *training* was based mostly on *practicing skills* - in the Viking days times that meant practicing with swords, spears and grappling - and *competition* in activities that were related to work or transportation, like lifting/ carrying, running, skiing, climbing and swimming. Sports were widely practiced and encouraged, especially those that involved weapons training and developing combat skills. This included spear and stone throwing, building and testing physical strength through wrestling, fist fighting, and stone lifting. Swimming was also a popular sport, as was mountain climbing. Agility and balance skills were built and tested by running and jumping.

The ancient Nordic way of physical activity ensured a balanced and functional fitness. Back in the days when manual labor was how you supported yourself and your family, which pretty much means until this last century, basic strength and endurance was a given. There was no need to design a progressive training program. If you could do more work or improve your skills you would, as this increased your security or even your chances of survival. These days however, it seems that the most important skills are practiced using only small gadgets. Survival is secured if you know how to operate a microwave oven or swipe a credit card.

Nonetheless, some of the Viking attitude has survived in the Nordic Countries through the last millennium: The love of the great outdoors and sports or activities that utilize the natural environment is still a considerable part of the culture, as is the prevalent DIY attitude, also when it comes to exercise or manual labor. As you may recall, the Nordics, i.e. Norway, Sweden, Denmark, Iceland and Finland, typically rank at the very top of international health and wellness statistics. They must be doing something right, although in fairness there could be a tiny bias here since the author is originally Norwegian. Yet even in these countries, the emergence of a less active lifestyle through the past few decades has led to a significant decline in physical ability. In short, we are sitting around way too much. The question is: How can we, as modern-day office workers and couch potatoes, recapture some of that brute strength and endurance of the old-time farmers and seafarers and avoid breaking down prematurely?

The System

Enter the Nordic Method. This training system is based on the way exercise has been done in the Nordic Countries in the past century: Community-based, often led by non-professional enthusiasts, and focused on functional strength and conditioning training. This is not an attempt at replicating what the ancient Vikings did, although that could potentially be a lot of fun. The objective is rather to bring us back to a state of general physical fitness that will allow such playful competitiveness.

The Nordic Method is built around a few foundational beliefs:

- Training should make you healthier, more functional and increase your overall fitness. A possible exception is if you're training for extremely high performance in a competitive sport, in which case you might accept some imbalance in your training.

- Training should, without significant risk of injury, prepare you to safely and competently overcome the challenges you may meet in everyday life, such as picking up and carrying a child, lift a suitcase into the overhead compartment, push a loaded wheelbarrow, carry heavy grocery bags, get your loved ones out of a burning building, or – most dangerous of all - sit in an office chair all day.

- Strength comes first, regardless of your ultimate goal, even if it's losing weight or being able to run a marathon. Strength training will make you move more efficiently. It will boost your metabolism dramatically, fostering sustained changes to your body composition. A well-balanced strength-training program will also even out joint misalignments, a common source of injury e.g. in runners.

- To control external objects you must first be able to control your own body, i.e. the system must emphasize using your own bodyweight as resistance, overcoming the pull of gravity in a controlled manner. Implicitly, you don't need a lot of fancy gadgets to work out.

- When external resistance is used, it should mimic real-life challenges such as physical labor. The training must therefore be functional rather than muscle isolating, i.e. primarily utilizing full body or multi-joint movements. When a particular body part is under heavy load, the rigid framework of the rest of body should support it, not external objects.

- External resistance loads should be in the range most commonly encountered in everyday life, i.e. up to about your own bodyweight. The exception is some pushing and pulling motions, where the weight of the object could be considerably higher if you're working to overcome frictional forces and inertia rather than gravity, e.g. when pushing a car.

- Time is precious. Any training system should be designed to give maximum benefit with minimum time expenditure.

- Most things (with a few notable exceptions) are better when done in the company of other people. This includes exercising, and the program should thus be easy to adapt for communal workouts.

If you have picked up this book and read this far, chances are you're already working out but are looking for a different take on your workouts. Or you haven't been working out in a while and are motivated to make a lasting change to your fitness level or physique. Regardless of motivation, the sad truth is that many people don't achieve their fitness goals. The missing link is often in the distinction between workout and training: A workout can take many different forms, and if you've built up a sweat and feel good afterwards, chances are you'll be quite satisfied with yourself. After a while, though, this won't necessarily result in much progress. The body is very good at adapting to new circumstances, and unless we keep on challenging ourselves, it will simply settle into a new comfort zone.

Training, on the other hand, is a number of workouts with progressive levels of difficulty, designed to achieve a goal of some sort. Hence a training program or workout system is needed, i.e. a progressive sequence of workouts that will continue to challenge the body to adapt to new and more demanding circumstances, and that is precisely what the Nordic Method is. Constantly challenging yourself is hard, but well worth the effort.

In this book, you'll find a compilation of 150 workouts, enough to last a full year for most people. The program has been organized into 3 workouts per week, whereof 2 are considered essential for your progress. If you stick to it, the Nordic Method program will make you more aligned, less prone to injury, stronger, leaner, and tougher; and it will increase your stamina and work capacity. It is however not designed to add much muscle mass or make you run a faster 10k or marathon, although this could be a side effect for some, depending on the starting point. If one of those is your main goal, or you're training for sports-specific performance, you may consider using parts of this program as an addition to your specific training, rather than as the mainstay. With slight modifications, such as increasing the level of difficulty on some of the bodyweight moves or using heavier loads where external resistance is required, this program can be recycled and reused for years.

A Not-So-Brief Q&A Session

What is the Nordic Method?

The Nordic Method is a functional strength and conditioning workout system. It was conceived as a way for communities or groups of friends to work out together with very little equipment, but can just as well be used by individuals. The program comprises 150 workouts in total, a full year's worth, designed to progressively increase your functionality, strength and stamina. It has also been designed as a mega-cycle, meaning that with some minor adjustments, the program can be re-used year upon year.

Functional strength, you say? What does that mean, exactly?

Functional exercise has become a ridiculously overused term in the fitness industry, so perhaps we should first determine what it is not. For several decades, the fitness industry propagated the idea that in order to effectively train strength, you must try to isolate each muscle as much as possible. You may have heard exercises explained along the lines of "preacher curls will enhance the biceps peak". It is mostly a load of nonsense. The point is: Although potentially effective from an aesthetic standpoint, isolating a specific muscle is rarely functional. The body is designed to work as a whole, and functional training must therefore take an holistic approach, nurturing movement patterns and function rather than individual muscle growth and aesthetics. The concept of isolation is something that originated in bodybuilding, and in the context of that sport it makes perfect sense: To accurately shape your physique to aesthetic perfection, you must be able to control the shape of each individual muscle to the minute detail. However, there is a catch. Without a rock-solid foundation and a deep understanding of what you're doing, this strategy does not work all that well.

All the groundbreaking pioneers from the Golden Age of bodybuilding – Joe Weider, Arnold Schwarzenegger, Frank Zane, Dave Draper, and the rest – knew that you needed a really good foundation in the big compound lifts, i.e. deadlifts, squats and presses. These big lifts are inherently functional: They develop strength in fundamental, multi-joint movements, and they develop considerable muscle mass if you go at it heavy and hard. When this foundation was in place, a bodybuilder could spend time fine-tuning the precise shape of individual muscles using isolation exercises. Sadly, somewhere along the way, it seems the knowledge that functional strength is the basis for everything got lost to the mainstream consciousness. Fitness industry companies latched on to the achievements of the Golden Age heroes and started making equipment that would mimic isolation exercises without requiring the strenuous, foundational work in the big lifts. Nowadays, most fitness facilities have a variety of complicated weight training machines that target and isolate specific muscles: Excessive use of such machines and equipment could make you *less* functional, create imbalances, and result in injury. Although possibly assisting in performing certain movements in a reasonably correct manner, machines also restrict your range of motion and deactivate the crucial supporting muscles that keep your joints in alignment. By the way, the same logic could be applied to the very monotonous movement patterns in some typical endurance sports, e.g. road race bicycling.

So let's be somewhat more specific: Functional training attempts to adapt or develop exercises that allow individuals to perform the activities of daily life more easily and without injuries. Functional training does not require a host of gadgets and equipment, but rather that you move in ways that mimic everyday challenges. Standing from a seated position, pulling your self up, throwing, running, picking things up and lifting them overhead - these are all functional movements. Although individual exercises will certainly work some body parts and motion patterns more than others, the whole body is typically involved in supporting that motion. This is a fundamental aspect of functional training. A functional fitness regimen, then, would be one that utilizes functional exercises to address and enhance our ability to successfully complete these types of everyday tasks.

What should a functional strength program look like, then?

According to the global depository of moderately curated facts, Wikipedia, a functional training program should be based on functional tasks directed toward everyday life activities. It should be *integrated*, i.e. include a variety of exercises that work on flexibility, core, balance, strength and power, focusing on multiple movement planes. It should be *progressive*, steadily increasing the difficulty of the task. Furthermore, a good program would need to be *periodized* to allow full development of different skills, mainly by training with distributed practice and varying the tasks, and repeated frequently with incorporated feedback following performance.

The best training programs are tailored to each individual, i.e. *individualized*. Any program must be specific to the goals of an individual, focusing on meaningful tasks. It must also be specific to the individual state of health, including presence or history of injury. An assessment should be performed to help guide exercise selection and training load. In addition to all this, a functional training program should ideally also use real life object manipulation in context-specific environments.

Cool. Does the Nordic Method cover all these points?

Yes - almost, but not entirely. It is indeed based primarily on functional tasks that mimic everyday activities. Or to put it differently: The exercises and workout structures are based on motion patterns rather than muscles or muscle group; e.g. lifting stuff off the ground, controlling the position of your body, or lifting loads overhead. This carries over well to everyday life.

It is also integrated, progressive, periodized, and repeated frequently. Given that this is not based on personal instruction, however, the performance feedback is intermittent. You will perform a benchmark test several times during the course of the program, and this will give you good indications of your success. Day-to-day feedback will largely be up to your own perceptiveness and that of your workout buddies.

The program is also standardized to some extent, which means that real-life object manipulation and context-specific environments are not available options unless you modify. The same goes for individualization: This will be up to you. For instance, you will find that the program indicates relative loads rather than specific loads, i.e. "heavy kettlebell" rather than "70-pound kettlebell". Since your capability is individual, so must the loads be – it is your job to learn to know yourself and adapt loads or specific exercise varieties to a suitably challenging level.

Who is the program for? Will it work for everyone?

It would be nice to say that it's for any and all, but that would be a somewhat ridiculous statement. It may be easier to tell you who it was originally made for: The first version of the Nordic Method program was put together for a group of friends who wanted to work out together in the parks of Silicon Valley. The program was hence designed to function well in a group setting with little available equipment. Most of the workouts can just as well be done on your own, though. The typical Nordic Method community member is within an age range from the late twenties to mid fifties. In California, the female-to-male ratio is 70/30, in Norway it is 40/60 – in other words, gender is irrelevant. Your results will depend on your starting point and how much effort you put into it. People with some past training experience, for instance former college athletes, tend to understand the requirements more easily and get results more quickly. Long-term however, consistency and effort yield the best results, regardless of starting point. But the bottom line is: You certainly don't need to be superhuman to do this. Normal is good enough.

Is there any chance I'll be injured?

Yes, any training program carries that risk. But if you're reasonably healthy and have no particular physical issues, it really isn't very likely. The Nordic Method program starts with fairly simple exercises and gradually evolves to more advanced movements and workouts, building on the work you've done. As long as you pay attention to how individual exercises should be performed and follow the progression of workouts without shopping around, you should be well prepared for the more complex parts of the program. There are nonetheless some risk factors to be aware of:

(1) Previous injuries. If you've had a traumatic injury in the past, especially joint- or back-related injuries, you need to be extra careful. The absence of pain is not necessarily a good indicator of function; it could be that you've simply learned how to avoid motion that may cause pain. You could still easily get re-injured if the joint function is still compromised. Start gently, slowly and with light loads for any exercise that involves the previously injured body part. Always start with your weak side and let that be the guide for how much you can do.

(2) False expectations. If you've been very active in the past, e.g. a competitive athlete, and you're now returning after a longer hiatus, you may suffer from a wrongful (I'll refrain from saying delusional) self-image. I certainly did. You may have a mental image of yourself doing quite spectacular things that you are no longer capable of and this will put you firmly in the risk-zone. Again, it's a good idea to start gently and probe your capabilities before pushing hard. If you've had some experience with barbell training, you should also be aware that kettlebells do not behave like barbells. The motion dynamics are quite different, so you cannot expect to be able to handle the same loads without preparation and practice.

(3) Competitiveness. Especially in combination with one or both of the previous points. You may be an outstanding golfer, soccer player, zumbaist, or whatever, but it really isn't the same. Let competitiveness fuel your motivation, but do not let it guide you when it comes to your exercise performance or choice of external loads. Never mind the damned Joneses. I'm not convinced that curiosity killed the cat, but competitiveness might have.

(4) Fast, heavy or complex exercises. Examples include sprinting, powerful jumps, and potentially heavy grinds like pull-ups, deadlifts or kettlebell presses. Such exercises require you to be well warmed up, ideally including a motion-specific warm-up. You'll also need to be extra focused on correct execution: If you find that your form is going downhill, stop what you're doing and rest.

(5) Insidious pain. Sometimes an injury can sneak up on you slowly, and these can turn out quite serious. It often starts as a dull ache that comes back every time you do specific exercises. After a while it can turn into chronic pain and be very difficult to get rid of. Pay attention to what your body is telling you: If you consistently get dull aches in the same spot, especially around the joints, it's typically an indication that you're doing something wrong. Most often, it'll be a minor error in the execution of an exercise that you do frequently – such as a small inward twist of the elbow when you do pull-ups, or one knee twisting a little when you squat. Over time it'll aggregate into an inflammation. Reassess often and try to capture these injuries before they take root. One additional thing: Many (not to say most) of us suffer from minor misalignments, such as a slight tilt to one side or a twist in the hips. This is typically brought on by sitting around too much, and is the result of permanent tightness in some muscles and too little tension in others. It is frequently a slight displacement of the hips, but that's not necessarily where people feel pain. The misalignment often shows up as a muscle knot somewhere else, for instance around the shoulder blade, the neck, or in the legs. It commonly occurs just on one side of the body. The Nordic Method program will take care of some misalignments, but probably not if it's severe. If you suspect that you may have a musculoskeletal misalignment, please go see an osteopath. Alternatively, you can do what I did: Read Pete Egoscue's *Health through Motion* (published by Harper Collins and available on Amazon), and do the prescribed exercises on your own. It works.

I don't want to bulk up. Will this make me big?

No, it will not. However, muscular development depends to some extent on your starting point. If you have not done any significant strength training in the past, you may growth of some muscle groups. For most people though, the end result tends to be increased muscle density and definition, generally having a slimming effect. For significant muscle growth to occur, you would need heavier loads and a lot more workouts with exercises done to failure, i.e. complete muscle fatigue. That said, most people find that the upper body becomes more muscled with much better muscle definition, especially around the shoulder area.

I really want to bulk up. Will this make me big?

No, it will not. However, muscular development depends to some extent on your starting point. If you have not done any significant strength training in the past, or if your strength training has been imbalanced, you may experience growth of some muscle groups. For most people though, the end result tends to be increased muscle density and definition, generally having a slimming effect. A proper muscle-building program would require heavier loads and more sets performed to full muscle fatigue. That said, the Nordic Method workout system will provide an excellent *foundation* for hypertrophic training, i.e. training designed specifically to enhance muscle growth. It will give you a well-balanced physique, improved joint alignment, much-improved strength endurance, better neuro-muscular activation, and stronger joints and ligaments. All of this will serve you well if you decide to embark on a true muscle-building program.

Should I perhaps go on a diet?

Don't. Just… don't. What I mean is, you should not base your food intake on an unsustainable model, and that's precisely what a classic diet is. Changing your overall dietary regime to something better could be a good idea, but you need to think *permanent and sustainable* change. I'm not saying that you should never diet; after all, most major religions have the concept of fasting baked into them, and there could be a reason for that. As such, something like a week of fresh-vegetables-and-water-only each year may not be such a bad idea. But it's our general eating habits and basic food intake that needs to be of the best possible quality. When it is, no dieting should be needed. A simple strategy is to try to eat more of the good stuff. Eventually it'll crowd out the bad stuff. I'm sure you have pretty good idea of what belongs in those categories.

I'm certainly no nutritionist, so I'll keep this fairly short. My personal opinion – and consequently how I practice this myself – is based on a few very simple rules:

1. Eat real food. In other words, stick mainly to food items that carry no label, such as unprocessed fish, meat, vegetables, fruits, seeds and nuts. If there is a label, be very skeptical to anything that lists more than 6 ingredients. If it sounds like a chemical it probably is and shouldn't be eaten.

2. If it has a shelf life of more than a week or two, it's not food. Exception: Dry goods that comply with Rule # 1.

3. Make your own meals. It takes less than 10 minutes to fry a steak or boil an egg. It takes less than a minute to peel and eat a banana. Why choose a premade meal full of dubious ingredients to be nuked in the microwave? If you eat out, choose restaurants where people care about the food.

4. Drink water, and only that, several times a day. Exceptions: A couple of cups of coffee or tea per day. And the occasional glass of wine, obviously.

5. Refined sugar is a poison and more addictive than cocaine. High fructose corn syrup is worse. Treat it accordingly. Many industrially processed foods will have high sugar content and should be avoided. If in doubt, see Rule #1.

6. Go easy on bread and dairy. See Rules #1 and #2 for guidance.

7. Always eat breakfast. No exceptions.

It's all well with this strength stuff, but shouldn't we be doing some cardio?

Right. Well, it's a little complicated. Cardio is an abbreviated term used for cardio-vascular or cardio-respiratory capacity training, in other words increasing the work capacity of the heart and respiratory system. This can be achieved in a number of ways, also with a program that is mostly focused on strength. Sadly, the impression that strength training results in no "cardio" development seems to have stuck. Admittedly, it may be true for the training of *absolute* strength, e.g. some of the maximum load training a world-class powerlifter would do, such as deadlifting 900 pounds, although I think you'd be surprised at the work capacity these people have. It can also be true for neuro-muscular stimulation training or technique work, i.e. training designed to increase the number of neural connections to your muscle tissue and specific neural pathways. However, for many varieties of moderate to high rep strength training, it certainly is not.

Most people use the term "cardio" to mean "long-lasting, slow, semi-steady state cardio-vascular work", i.e. maintaining an elevated heart rate, typically in the 130-150 beats per minute (bpm) range, for a long time (hours). To achieve this, you would need to choose an activity where the energy expenditure per time unit is moderate and fairly consistent, such as jogging or road biking. This strategy is efficient for increasing the body's capability to distribute the inhaled oxygen. The challenge with some of these typical "cardio" exercises is that they often have quite monotonous motion patterns – biking in particular – and since the body is really good at adapting, it'll quickly try to make these patterns more efficient. In other words, it'll seek to reduce the energy spent doing it.

It is, however, not the only way to train cardio-vascular capacity, nor necessarily the most efficient one. You typically get the most bang for the buck from training that briefly pushes the heart rate very high, say 180bpm, followed by an active rest period that is just sufficient to allow the heart rate to come back down and your muscles to be oxygenated. An excellent way to achieve this is by doing interval training, in other words going very hard at something for a brief period of time (tens of seconds to a few minutes), then resting or doing a less strenuous activity for a similar period of time. The activities should have high expenditure of energy, such as lifting heavy objects or sprinting. Circuit training is one good example, and we'll be doing a lot of that. I once tried squatting with a 225-pound bar for 50 reps without putting the bar down. Give it a try. Afterwards we can discuss how there is "no cardio" in strength training. To stop me blabbering about this, please accept the following: It's baked into the program, to a reasonable degree. If you need more, feel free to add some in.

So, is the Nordic Method, like, the Ultimate Program?

Ummm… no. No it is not. Such a thing is quite hard to come by. The ultimate program would be specifically tailored to your goals, your genetics and your condition. It would also be adjusted on a daily basis, not to say in real time, depending on how you respond to the training, taking into account any injuries past and present, and even external factors in your life such as sleep; what you've eaten and how much; your emotional state; work; travel; and so on and so forth. That's to some extent how things work for the most accomplished professional athletes with huge support organizations. The Nordic Method cannot provide this kind of detailed adaptation to your individual needs, unfortunately. The program is however a reasonable approximation to something that works for well for most people.

How long does each workout take?

Mostly about an hour or less, including warm-up.

Should I stick to the program exactly as written?

Not necessarily. In fact, I expect you not to. The program is but a suggestion, albeit a strong one, and you must always pay attention to what your body is telling you. If you're having a really bad day, take it a little easy and feel free to skip a couple of exercises. If you're having a great day, go a little heavier or add in something extra. Are your shoulders tense and sore after carrying a sick child all night? Maybe you should do lightweight overhead presses even if the program indicates heavy loads. Are you training for something particular, like totally dominating the annual corporate 10k-run? Skip one of the three weekly workouts from this program for a while and add in two days of running. Is the coming week full of logistical insanity? Train a little if and when you can, then return with a vengeance next week. It's not carved in stone. But do try to stick to the week-by-week progression of workouts; it's set up that way for a reason. And do your very best to stay consistent with your training.

I want additional exercise. What should it be?

What do you enjoy? If you think it's fun, go ahead and do it! There are some activities that are complementary to the Nordic Method program and that I generally recommend based on their being beneficial from a functional perspective. These include: Hiking (off trail if possible); Running (sprint intervals or trail); Basketball; Cross-country skiing; Swimming; Dancing (especially street or freestyle); Martial arts; and Yoga. Do you have very specific goals? Do that.

Equipment

You really don't need much equipment to go ahead with the Nordic Method: More than anything else the program relies on the resistance provided by your own bodyweight. Most of what we do only requires a suitable place to work out, and a few objects to provide some added resistance. What you need to get started is this:

- One kettlebell for the first few months, later one or preferably two heavier kettlebells.
- Access to a pull-up bar and playground swings, alternatively gymnastic rings or adjustable TRX straps.
- Something stable and solid to step and jump onto, approximately 20-24" height; e.g. a box, bench or low wall.
- A sturdy towing rope or similar.
- Nice to have: A large, soft, medicine ball (5-10kg or 10-25lbs).
- Nice to have: Rubber resistance bands.
- Nice to have: A sledgehammer.

Kettlebells are essentially cannon balls with handles. They originated in Russia centuries ago, where farmers would use them to weigh down tarpaulins that covered piles of grain in the fields. As it is with these things, the young men started competing amongst themselves about who could lift the heaviest one overhead, or swing it the most times in a row. Since then, kettlebell training has been used extensively in Russia for strength and conditioning, among athletes, strongmen and military alike. It is a supremely effective training tool, improving both strength, endurance, flexibility, explosiveness, and balance.

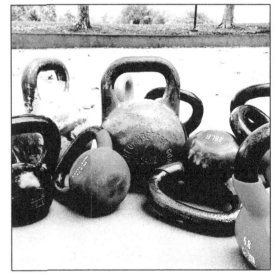

Ideally, you should have a few different kettlebells for different types of exercises, at least a light bell for pressing and some complicated exercises, and a heavier bell for squats and swings. The perfect kit would be to have two each of a light, a medium and a heavy kettlebell: 8, 12, and 16kg (15/ 25/ 35lbs) for ladies; 12, 16, and 24kg (25/ 35/ 50lbs) for guys.

However, good kettlebells can be quite costly, and it may be prudent to start out with just one. If so, the starting weight for men is normally 12kg (25lbs) if you have limited experience with strength training, and 16kg (35lbs) if you have done a quite a bit of strength work and kept it up. For women, the equivalent would be 8kg (15lbs) or 12kg (25lbs). You could go lighter, but should then be prepared to get yourself a heavier bell after a few weeks of kettlebell training. A good, individual test is to try pressing the bell overhead (see exercise [A14] KB Press in the chapter on Exercises); if you can do 5-8 presses, the weight is about right for you.

There are a number of different companies offering kettlebells, and you'll find some in most major sports equipment stores. Go for one that is all steel; the plastic ones have more limited application, e.g. cannot be tossed or dragged. If you are determined to include kettlebells as a central part of your workout program, and if you have the financial means, I recommend considering a somewhat more costly competition kettlebell, e.g. by Perform Better or Rage Fitness. You'll be looking at roughly 80-100 $ apiece, depending on the size – about twice the price of simpler kettlebells. The competition kettlebell have the benefit of being larger, i.e. the diameter is greater and will not hurt (as much) when you rack them against your arms; better quality and durability; and they are also of uniform size regardless of weight, i.e. you will not have to modify your technique as you work with different weights.

Ropes are extremely useful for a number of different pulling exercises, such as inverted rows, buddy pulls and pull-ups. Some of this can of course be done with gymnastic rings or TRX straps instead, if you have that. If you do get a rope, it needs to be thick enough that it's reasonably comfortable to hold onto; that generally means at least 1 inch. It should also be resilient to fraying – the rope will suffer some hard use. We recommend a good sturdy towing rope or towing slings, available from any hardware store.

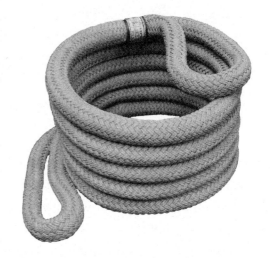

Resistance bands are very convenient, both to reduce resistance in the standard bodyweight exercises, and for adding extra resistance to those if you need it. They can be a little pricey though, typically in the range of 25 – 60 US$. Nonetheless, after a few experiences that could have turned really ugly – involuntary sterilization comes to mind – it is recommended that you consider resistance bands that are of a good, durable quality. The types that look like ridiculously oversized household rubber bands are the most versatile. The types that are thin, flimsy straps are not quite as useful, and tend to tear along the edges. There are numerous vendors on Amazon that deliver good quality bands, such as Serious Steel, WODfitters, Y-SportLive, Viking Strong and Rage Fitness.

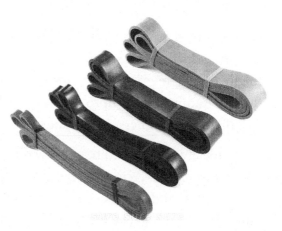

Testing

If you want to know how you're doing, you need to know where you are, where you've been, and where you're going. For this very reason we perform progress tests. It really isn't a major part of the program: There is only one test, and we do it six times in total through the year. It is important though.

Our primary test is called the **Bodyweight 500**, or **BW500** for short. As you might have surmised, it consists of exercises with your own bodyweight as resistance only. There are seven different exercises, and you'll do a total of 500 repetitions. The sequence is as follows:

> 25 repetitions of Inverted Rows.
>
> 50 repetitions of Burpees.
>
> 50 repetitions of Push-Ups.
>
> 100 repetitions of Air Squats.
>
> 100 repetitions of Mountain Climbers (50 each side).
>
> 100 repetitions of Glute Bridges.
>
> 50 repetitions of Rower Sit-Ups.
>
> 25 repetitions of Inverted Rows.

The exercises must be performed in this order, i.e. all repetitions of one exercise must be completed before you move on to the next. You may take a break whenever you like for as long as you like, but the objective is to complete everything, all 500 repetitions, in as little time as possible. This will give you a general indication of your combined strength endurance and cardio-respiratory conditioning. People often struggle with the strength endurance part at first; it is easy to "burn out", especially on the upper body exercises (Push-Ups and Inverted Rows). Just completing a single repetition of each of these can be a challenge for many at first. Modifications of these two exercises are therefore allowed if you're unable to do more than 5 consecutive repetitions of either one, in which case you're encouraged to stick to that modification through the entire 6-test cycle for comparison purposes. When strength endurance improves, the limiting factor shifts to heart rate and breathing.

Note down your total time when you've completed the whole sequence, and compare your results the next time around. You should see significant progress through the year, provided that you've put some serious effort into the workouts. Initially, people tend to get through the Bodyweight 500 in around 35 minutes. Those who have done similar training in the past could start out below 25 minutes. During the course of the Nordic Method program, test times normally drop approximately 10 minutes; a little more if initial test times were in the high end, less if they were below 25 minutes. The best test times recorded so far have been around 13 minutes. That's the same as doing almost 39 repetitions every minute on average, or about 1.6 seconds per repetition. In other words there really isn't much time left for rest.

What's the limit for performance on the BW500 test? Hard to tell, but my best guess is around 12 minutes. At that point you'll be going at a steady rate of less than 1.5 seconds per repetition, and that's about as fast as you can execute most of these exercises with good form. If you reach this level, put on a weight vest. Or find yourself another test to measure your continued progress: There are some workouts in the final third of the Nordic Method program that could serve as tests: Number 112, 143 and 146 would be good candidates. If the notes say "AQAP" (i.e. As Quickly As Possible) for the whole workout, it's an indication that you could time that program and use it for testing. That'll be up to you, though.

Program Layout

The Nordic Method program is loosely structured into 10 phases, each with a particular focus and lasting 5 weeks. These are as follows:

(1) Weeks 1-5 (workouts 1-15):
Introduction of basic exercises. Circuit training for fundamental conditioning.

(2) Weeks 6-10 (workouts 16-30):
Increased conditioning focus. Introduction of kettlebell exercises and running.

(3) Weeks 11-15 (workouts 31-45):
Short cycle conditioning. Advanced kettlebell complexes.

(4) Weeks 16-20 (workouts 46-60):
Increased variety of exercises. Introduction to heavy conditioning.

(5) Weeks 21-25 (workouts 61-75):
Heavy conditioning 1: Harder exercises, bodyweight/kettlebell combination programs.

(6) Weeks 26-30 (workouts 76-90):
Heavy conditioning 2: Harder exercises, bodyweight/kettlebell combination programs.

(7) Weeks 31-35 (workouts 91-105):
Consolidation. Slightly less demanding programs, few new exercises.

(8) Weeks 36-40 (workouts 106-120):
Heavy conditioning 3: Bodyweight/ kettlebell combination programs.

(9) Weeks 41-45 (workouts 121-135):
Consolidation, repetition, and variety challenges.

(10) Weeks 46-50 (workouts 136-150):
Consolidation, repetition, and variety challenges.

It's not entirely clear-cut: The predominant focus areas are typically introduced in the period preceding the main phase and will also flow into the subsequent period before fading out. The overall progression is important, though. Ideally, you should stick to the week-by-week layout – at least through Phase 6. In phases 9 and 10 you can freely shop around if you feel like it.

Using the Program

Chances are that parts of the following will be an over-simplification for some people, but I'd be grateful if you'd indulge me and skim through. An important note: There are some workouts in the first 10 weeks of the program that are marked "Advanced". These are intended for people who have already completed a full year's cycle and they comprise exercises that new trainees are not prepared for.

The workouts in Chapter 3 are presented as tables, detailing which exercises should be done, how much and in which order, the amount rest between the sets, and other particulars related to performing the exercises. As might be expected, you should start at the top of the table and work your way down. There is a lot of information packed into these tables, and it may require some background information to decipher it. From left to right, the columns are as follows:

M	R	Exercise	Sets	Reps	Rest	Notes
(1) Mode	(2) Rounds	(3)	(4)	(5)	(6)	(7)

(1) MODE

The Mode indicates *how* the workout should be performed, i.e. the manner in which the different exercises follow each other. The size of the merged box shows which exercises should be included in that particular mode. There are four (4) different modes in use:

Sequence

A sequence is a number of exercises performed in the order listed for the indicated number of sets, i.e. Exercise A – B – C – D – E, in that order. Repeat the sequence for the indicated number of rounds.

Circuit

A Circuit is quite similar to a Sequence, except that the you could start anywhere in the listed sequence. In other words, you could to the exercises in the order D – E – A – B – C, if needed. This is a practical way of arranging things if the workout is done in a group and you are limited on equipment. The order of exercises could be re-arranged too, if it works better for your particular workout location, but should ideally be kept close to the original.

Superset

A Superset is essentially a very short sequence with only two exercises. You'll typically alternate between the two each set.

Standalone

If nothing is written in the two left-hand columns, the exercise is a standalone, i.e. you'll perform all the prescribed sets of this exercise before moving on to the next.

(2) ROUNDS

The Rounds column shows the number of times you should perform a Sequence, Circuit or Superset. You will occasionally encounter the term AMRAP, meaning 'As Many Rounds As Possible'. If so, you'll also find a notation on the far right stating how long you should keep going, e.g. 20 minutes. In practical terms you would then do as many rounds as you can manage in 20 minutes and you'd adjust the rest periods according to your current condition and how tough you'd like it to be.

(3) EXERCISE

Names the exercises to be performed. These exercises are all described in Chapter 4. Each exercise will also have a reference number attached to the name, e.g. [A14] KB Press. This is done to make it easier to find a particular exercise in the reference chapter – they are not organized alphabetically. The exercises are rather grouped together by type, and then roughly sorted by how strenuous or complicated they are, from easiest to hardest.

You will also note that in some workout tables, the name of one or more exercises will be written in **bold letters**: This indicates the first time that that particular exercise is introduced. The exception to this rule is exercises that are listed in the workouts marked with "Advanced" in the first ten weeks. These workouts are intended only for trainees who have already done a full year of Nordic Method and thus know all the exercises.

(4) SETS

A Set is several repetitions of the same exercise performed without rest. The Sets column will show the number of Sets of a particular exercise to be performed before you move on. When you're done with a Set, you rest and repeat for the prescribed number, or move on to the next exercise.

The suffix "ea." means that you should do the prescribed number of sets <u>each side.</u> For instance: If you're doing Kettlebell Presses and the Sets column reads "2 ea.", it means that you should do two sets on the right hand side, and two sets on the left-hand side.

(5) REPS

Reps is short for Repetitions. One repetition is a particular Exercise done in the prescribed manner for a single execution. The Reps column shows the number of repetitions to be performed in each Set. In the modes Circuit and Sequence you will often see something like "20s/set"; this means each Set shall last for 20 seconds, and in that time you do as many repetitions with good form as you can manage.

You will also encounter the acronym AMRAP, meaning As Many Repetitions As Possible; which would mean, "Do as many as you can without stopping". Likewise, you may see the term ALAP, As Long As Possible. This is sometimes used if you should hold a static position for as long as you can. In some cases there will be a percentage indicator, e.g. "50%', meaning that you should make an estimate of the maximum repetitions you could do in one go, and then do half of that.

There are some workouts in the program where you'll see something like "$1a_19d_11$". This is a shorthand way of writing, "Start with 1 rep, then add 1 rep each set until you reach 9, whereupon you decrease 1 rep each set until you're back at 1 rep". Or in numbers: 1, 2, 3, 4, 5, 6, 7, 8, 9, 8, 7, 6, 5, 4, 3, 2, 1. Or how about this one: "$10d_11$". That'll be "start with 10 reps on the first set, then decrease one rep per set until you reach 1 rep". One additional example: "$1a_1Max$". Got it? Oh well, it is "start with 1 rep, then add one rep per set until you reach your maximum". You'll figure it out for sure.

By the way: We always count every rep. In other words, if it's an exercise where you switch sides, one left and one right is counted as 2 reps.

(6) REST

In general, the rest column will state the length of the rest period after each Set or Round, in seconds or minutes. There are some exceptions, though:

- *Brief* - means that it's up to you, but try to keep it to a few seconds at most.
- *n/a* – Not Applicable. Alas! there will be no rest for the wicked. Or very little, at least. Indicates that you should keep the rest breaks as short as you possibly can.
- *As req.* - As Required. In other words, it's up to you. Resume when ready, within reason. Next year would be stretching it a bit too far.
- *S/U* - Stand Up between sets, but nothing more. Get back down there and barge on.
- *=walk* – walk back to start.

(7) NOTES

This column provides supplementary directions to how an exercise or a training mode should be performed, e.g. how large the external resistance load should be (in relative terms), or if you should do the exercise faster or slower than normal. I'm sure you'll figure out most of it.

Some examples:

- *1KB/2KB* – Indicates if you should use one or two kettlebells.

- *10-count* – Move slowly on each repetition, counting to 10, i.e. roughly 1 rep./10 sec.

- *Alt. ea.* – Alternate each rep, i.e. change sides.

- *Alt./set* – Alternate each set, i.e. change sides.

- *AMRAP* – As many repetitions or rounds as possible in the allotted time.

- *AQAP* – As quickly as possible.

- *Light* – Use a light-weight kettlebell (lighter than normal) if you have one.

- *Medium* – Use your standard kettlebell.

- *Heavy* – Use a heavier-than-normal kettlebell if you have one.

- *X-Heavy* – Use a really challenging kettlebell if you have one.

- *Opt.* – Optional. For instance, add some kettlebells for extra resistance or skip the rest period.

- *Hold* – Hold tension for the indicated length of time each repetition.

- *Mod. as req.* – Modify as required. In other words, choose an easier version of the exercise if you need to.

- *Tabata* – The Tabata interval protocol, 8x20 seconds work with 10 seconds rest between the sets.

- *Until failure* – Continue until you can no longer do an additional repetition with decent form.

WEEK 3

#007 ☆ BW Conditioning

M	R	Exercise	Sets	Reps	Rest	Note
CIRCUIT	2	B03 **Seated Band Row**	2	15s each set	15s/ set, +1min/ round	Optional: One additional round.
		D12 Burpee	2			
		A03 **Half Push-Up**	2			
		C03 Air Squat	2			
		D02 **Shuffle Jump**	2			
		F06 Glute Bridge	2			
		E14 Rower Sit-Up	2			

#008 ☆ Circuit No. 1

M	R	Exercise	Sets	Reps	Rest	Note
CIRCUIT	2	C05 **Hindu Squat**	2	20s each set	20s/ set, +2min/ round	Optional: Less or no rest between sets of the same exercise.
		B02 Superman Row	2			
		A17 Seated Dips	2			
		C14 Step-Up	1 ea.			
		E09 Crunch	2			
		B01 Bat Wings	2			
		C02 Air Bench	2			
		F05 Straight Bridge, Static	2			
		E02 Plank	2			
		E04 Side Plank	1 ea.			
		F03 Down Dog / Up Dog	2			

#009 ✋ Advanced

M	R	Exercise	Sets	Reps	Rest	Note
SEQUENCE	2	B04 Standing Band Row	2	10	20s/ set, +1min/ round	Strength exercises can be done as supersets w/10s rest.
		E18 KB Russian Twist	2	10		
		G15 Run	1	~100m		
		C12 Sk8 Squat	2	10		
		D05 Vertical Frog Jump	2	10		
		G15 Run	1	~100m		
		A01 Band Push	2	10		
		F15 KB H2H Swing	2	10		

WEEK 4

#010 ☆ BW Conditioning

M	R	Exercise	Sets	Reps	Rest	Note
CIRCUIT	5	B08 Inverted Row	1	20s each set	20s/ set, +1min/ round	Mod. as req.
		D04 **Kick-Back Jump**	1			
		A01 **Band Push**	1			
		C03 Air Squat	1			
		E08 Everest Mtn. Climber	1			
		F08 **SL Glute Bridge, R**	1			
		F08 SL Glute Bridge, L	1			
		E11 **Reverse Crunch**	1			

#011 ☆ Circuit No. 1

M	R	Exercise	Sets	Reps	Rest	Note
CIRCUIT	2	F13 **KB 2h Swing**	2	20s each set	20s/ set, +2min/ round	Optional: Less or no rest between sets of the same exercise.
		C05 Hindu Squat	2			
		B02 Superman Row	2			
		A17 Seated Dips	2			
		C14 Step-Up	1 ea.			
		E19 **Seated Leg Raise**	2			
		A02 **Scapular Push-Up**	2			
		C02 Air Bench	2			
		F05 Straight Bridge, Static	2			
		E02 Plank	2			
		E04 Side Plank	1 ea.			
		F03 Down Dog / Up Dog	2			

#012 ✋ Advanced

M	R	Exercise	Sets	Reps	Rest	Note
		B13 Pull-Up	6	30%	45s	Mod. as req.
SEQ.	5	F13 KB 2h Swing	1	15s each	1min/ round	
		F14 KB 1h Swing, R	1			
		F14 KB 1h Swing, L	1			
		F15 KB H2H Swing	1			
		A06 Push-Up	1	AMRAP	1min	
		C04 Squat Jump	8	20s	10s	Tabata

WEEK 5

#013 ☆ BW Conditioning

M	R	Exercise	Sets	Reps	Rest	Note
CIRCUIT	2	B03 Seated Band Row	2	20s	20s, +2min/ round	Mod. as req.
		D12 Burpee	2	20s		
		A03 Half Push-Up	2	20s		Mod. as req.
		C03 Air Squat	2	20s		
		E08 Everest Mtn. Climber	2	20s		
		F06 Glute Bridge	2	20s		
		E14 Rower Sit-Up	2	20s		

#014 ☆ Circuit No. 1

M	R	Exercise	Sets	Reps	Rest	Note
CIRCUIT	2	F13 KB 2h Swing	2	20s each set	15s/ set, +90s/ round	Optional: Less or no rest between sets of the same exercise.
		C05 Hindu Squat	2			
		B02 Superman Row	2			
		A17 Seated Dips	2			
		C14 Step-Up	1 ea.			
		E19 Seated Leg Raise	2			
		A02 Scapular Push-Up	2			
		C02 Air Bench	2			
		F05 Straight Bridge, Static	2			
		E02 Plank	2			
		E04 Side Plank	1 ea.			
		F03 Down Dog / Up Dog	2			

#015 ✋ Advanced

M	R	Exercise	Sets	Reps	Rest	Note
		E27 KB Turkish Get-Up	n/a	10min	Brief	Alt. ea.
SEQUENCE	2	C15 Step-Up Jump	1	20s each	10s/ set, +1min/ round	
		F13 KB 2h Swing	1			
		A08 Diamond Push-Up	1			
		F13 KB 2h Swing	1			
		C04 Squat Jump	1			
		F13 KB 2h Swing	1			
		E09 Crunch	1			Fast
		F13 KB 2h Swing	1			

WEEK 6

#016 ☆ TEST, The BW500

M	R	Exercise	Sets	Reps	Rest	Note
		ᴮ⁰⁸ Inverted Row	As req.	25		
		ᴰ¹² Burpee	As req.	50		
		ᴬ⁰⁶ Push-Up	As req.	50		AQAP
		ᶜ⁰³ Air Squat	As req.	100	As req.	
		ᴱ⁰⁸ Everest Mtn. Climber	As req.	100		For
		ᶠ⁰⁶ Glute Bridge	As req.	100		total time
		ᴱ¹⁴ Rower Sit-Up	As req.	50		
		ᴮ⁰⁸ Inverted Row	As req.	25		

#017 ☆ Circuit No. 2

M	R	Exercise	Sets	Reps	Rest	Note
		ᶠ¹⁷ **KB Clean**	5 ea.	5 ea.	20s ea.	Focus on form
CIRCUIT	2	ᶠ¹⁴ **KB 1h Swing**	1 ea.			
		ᴮ⁰⁵ **KB Supported Row**	1 ea.			
		ᶜ¹⁷ **Bwd Lunge**	1 ea.	30s each set	20s/ set, +2min/ round	
		ᶠ⁰⁴ **Bird Dog**	1 ea.			
		ᶠ⁰² **Dirty Dog**	1 ea.			
		ᴰ⁰¹ **Jumping Jack**	2			
		ᴬ⁰¹ **Band Push**	2			
		ᴱ¹² **Unicycle Crunch**	1 ea.			

#018 ✋ Advanced (KB Complex No. 1)

M	R	Exercise	Sets	Reps	Rest	Note
SEQ.	12	ᶠ¹⁸ KB Clean & Press, R	1	5	None/ set, 1min/ round	
		ᶜ¹⁹ KB OH Bwd Lun. R	1	5		
		ᶠ¹⁸ KB Clean & Press, L	1	5		
		ᶜ¹⁹ KB OH Bwd Lun. L	1	5		
		ᶠ¹³ KB 2h Swing	1	10		

WEEK 7

#019 ☆ BW Short Cycle

M	R	Exercise	Sets	Reps	Rest	Note
CIRC.	17	B08 Inverted Row	1	$1a_19d_11$	Brief/ set, 20-60s/ round	Pyramid: Ascending sets, then descending
		A02 Scapular Push-Up	1	$1a_19d_11$		
		E13 **Bicycle Crunch**	1	$2a_218d_22$		
		C05 Hindu Squat	1	$2a_218d_22$		

#020 ☆ Circuit No. 2

M	R	Exercise	Sets	Reps	Rest	Note
		A14 **KB Press**	5 ea.	3 ea.	20s ea.	Focus on form
CIRCUIT	2	F17 KB Clean	2	30s each set	20s/ set, +2min/ round	
		F14 KB 1h Swing	1 ea.			
		B05 KB Supported Row	1 ea.			
		C16 **Static Lunge**	1 ea.			
		F04 Bird Dog	1 ea.			
		F02 Dirty Dog	1 ea.			
		D01 Jumping Jack	2			
		A01 Band Push	2			
		E12 Unicycle Crunch	1 ea.			

#021 ✌ Advanced

M	R	Exercise	Sets	Reps	Rest	Note
		C10 KB OH Squat	2 ea.	8 ea.	30s ea.	Medium
		E25 KB Turkish Sit-Up	3 ea.	8 ea.	30s ea.	Medium
		F20 KB Low Windmill	3 ea.	8 ea.	30s ea.	Medium
SEQ.	4	E05 X-Kick High Plank	1	30s each	30s/ round	
		E02 Plank	1			
		C08 KB H2H Sumo Squat	1			

WEEK 8

#022 ☆ BW & Run

M	R	Exercise	Sets	Reps	Rest	Note
SEQUENCE	2	B03 Seated Band Row	2	10	20s/ set, +1min/ round	Strength exercises can be done as supersets w/10s rest.
		A04 **Negative Push-Up**	2	10		
		G15 **Run**	1	~100m		
		E14 Rower Sit-Up	2	10		
		C12 **Sk8 Squat**	2	10		
		G15 Run	1	~100m		
		F08 SL Glute Bridge	1 ea.	10		
		E17 **Russian Twist**	2	10		
		G15 Run	1	~100m		

#023 ☆ Circuit No. 2

M	R	Exercise	Sets	Reps	Rest	Note
		C07 **KB Goblet Squat**	5	6	30s	Focus on form
CIRCUIT	2	F18 **KB Clean & Press**	2	30s each set	20s/ set, +2min/ round	
		F14 KB 1h Swing	1 ea.			
		B05 KB Supported Row	1 ea.			
		C16 Static Lunge	1 ea.			
		F04 Bird Dog	1 ea.			
		F02 Dirty Dog	1 ea.			
		D01 Jumping Jack	2			
		A01 Band Push	2			
		E12 Unicycle Crunch	1 ea.			

#024 ✋ Advanced (Best Buddies)

M	R	Exercise	Sets	Reps	Rest	Note
SEQ.	4	G06 Wheelbarrow	1	20m each	1min each	
		G11 Buddy Carry	1			
		G12 Buddy Pull	1			
		G13 Reverse Buddy Pull	1			

WEEK 9

#025 ☆ BW Short Cycle

M	R	Exercise	Sets	Reps	Rest	Note
CIRC.	19	B08 Inverted Row	1	$1a_110d_11$	Brief/ set, 20-60s/ round	Pyramid: Ascending sets, then descending
		A02 Scapular Push-Up	1	$1a_110d_11$		
		E13 Bicycle Crunch	1	$2a_220d_22$		
		C05 Hindu Squat	1	$2a_220d_22$		

#026 ☆ Circuit No. 2

M	R	Exercise	Sets	Reps	Rest	Note
		F12 KB SL Deadlift	5 ea.	3 ea.	30s, 2nd	Focus on form
CIRCUIT	2	C07 KB Goblet Squat	2	30s each set	20s/ set, +2min/ round	
		F18 KB Clean & Press	1 ea.			
		F14 KB 1h Swing	1 ea.			
		B05 KB Supported Row	1 ea.			
		C17 Bwd Lunge	1 ea.			
		F04 Bird Dog	1 ea.			
		F02 Dirty Dog	1 ea.			
		D03 Zig Zag Jump	2			
		A01 Band Push	2			
		E10 Static Crunch	2			

#027 ✋ Advanced (Short Cycle AMRAP)

M	R	Exercise	Sets	Reps	Rest	Note
CIRC.	AMRAP	B12 Chin-Up	1	5	Brief	AMRAP 20min
		F16 KB High Swing	1	5		
		A18 Hanging Dips	1	5		
		D06 Vertical Jump	1	5		

WEEK 10

#028 ☆ BW & Run

M	R	Exercise	Sets	Reps	Rest	Note
SEQUENCE	2	B03 Seated Band Row	2	10	20s/ set, +1min/ round	Strength exercises can be done as supersets w/10s rest.
		A04 Negative Push-Up	2	10		
		G15 Run	1	~100m		
		E14 Rower Sit-Up	2	10		
		C12 Sk8 Squat	2	10		
		G15 Run	1	~100m		
		F08 SL Glute Bridge	1 ea.	10		
		E17 Russian Twist	2	10		
		G15 Run	1	~100m		

#029 ☆ Circuit No. 2

M	R	Exercise	Sets	Reps	Rest	Note
CIRCUIT	2	F12 KB SL Deadlift	1 ea.	30s each set	15s/ set, +2min/ round	
		C07 KB Goblet Squat	2			
		F18 KB Clean & Press	1 ea.			
		F14 KB 1h Swing	1 ea.			
		B05 KB Supported Row	1 ea.			
		C17 Bwd Lunge	1 ea.			
		F04 Bird Dog	1 ea.			
		F02 Dirty Dog	1 ea.			
		D03 Zig Zag Jump	2			
		A01 Band Push	2			
		E12 Unicycle Crunch	1 ea.			

#030 ✋ Advanced

M	R	Exercise	Sets	Reps	Rest	Note
CIRCUIT		A06 Push-Up	1	40s/ set	20s/ set, +2min/ round	5-count
		C20 KB Lunge Walk	1			2KB; Medium
		E25 KB Turkish Sit-Up	1			Alt. ea.
		F17 KB Clean	1			Med.; Alt. ea.
		D08 Box Jump	1			

WEEK 11

#031 ☆ BW & Run

M	R	Exercise	Sets	Reps	Rest	Note
		^{G15} Run	4	~100m	= walk	
SS	3	^{A06} Push-Up	1	AMRAP	1min	
		^{B08} Inverted Row	1	AMRAP	1min	
SS	2	^{E15} **Sit-Up**	1	20	1min	
		^{C12} Sk8 Squat	1	20	1min	
		^{G15} Run	4	~100m	= walk	

#032 ☆ KB Complex No. 1

M	R	Exercise	Sets	Reps	Rest	Note
SEQ.	12	^{F18} KB Clean & Press, R	1	3	None/ set, 1min/ round	
		^{C19} **KB OH Bwd Lun.** R	1	3		
		^{F18} KB Clean & Press, L	1	3		
		^{C19} KB OH Bwd Lun. L	1	3		
		^{F13} KB 2h Swing	1	10		

#033 – Circuit No. 3

M	R	Exercise	Sets	Reps	Rest	Note
CIRCUIT	2	^{F01} **Hurdles**	1 ea.	30s/ set	20s/ set, +2min/ round	Fast
		^{D05} **Vertical Frog Jump**	2			
		^{B02} Superman Row	2			
		^{D04} Kick-Back Jump	2			
		^{E03} **Low Plank**	2			30s or ALAP
		^{E06} **Bird Dog Plank**	2			Slow
		^{D02} Shuffle Jump	2			
		^{B04} **Standing Band Row**	2			
		^{C15} **Step-Up Jump**	2			

WEEK 12

#034 ☆ The Ministry of Funny Walks

M	R	Exercise	Sets	Reps	Rest	Note
SEQUENCE	3	G01 **Model Walk**	1	15-20m each	15-20s/ set, +1 min/ round	
		C18 **Lunge Walk**	1			
		G02 **Chaplin Walk**	1			
		G05 Bear Walk	1			
		D09 **Hzt Frog Jump**	1			
		G04 **Crab Walk**	1			
		D11 **Sprunglauf**	1			
		G06 **Wheelbarrow**	1			
		E16 **Sit-Up Twist**	3	8	30s	
		B02 Superman Row	3	15	30s	

#035 ☆ KB Complex No. 2

M	R	Exercise	Sets	Reps	Rest	Note
SEQ.	10	F18 KB Clean & Press, R	1	5	None/ set, 1min/ round	
		C09 **KB Front Squat**, R	1	5		
		F12 KB SL Deadlift, R	1	5		
		F18 KB Clean & Press, L	1	5		
		C09 KB Front Squat, L	1	5		
		F12 KB SL Deadlift, L	1	5		

#036 – BW & Run

M	R	Exercise	Sets	Reps	Rest	Note
SEQ.	10	A06 Push-Up	1	4	None/ set, 20s/ round	
		F03 Down Dog / Up Dog	1	4		
		E16 **Sit-Up Twist**	1	6		Alt. ea.
		C12 Sk8 Squat	1	6		Alt. ea.
		G15 Run	5	~100m	= walk	

WEEK 13

#037 ☆ Circuit No. 3

M	R	Exercise	Sets	Reps	Rest	Note
CIRCUIT	2	F01 Hurdles	1 ea.			Fast
		D05 Vertical Frog Jump	2			
		B02 Superman Row	2			
		D04 Kick-Back Jump	2		20s/ set, +2min/ round	
		E03 Low Plank	2	30s/ set		ALAP <30s
		E06 Bird Dog Plank	2			Slow
		D02 Shuffle Jump	2			
		B04 Standing Band Row	2			
		C15 Step-Up Jump	2			

#038 ☆ KB Complex No. 3

M	R	Exercise	Sets	Reps	Rest	Note
SEQUENCE	15	B07 **KB High Pull**, R	1	3		
		F17 KB Clean, R	1	1		
		A14 KB Press, R	1	3	None/ set, 1min/ round	
		C19 KB OH Bwd Lun. R	1	3		
		B07 KB High Pull, L	1	3		
		F17 KB Clean, L	1	1		
		A14 KB Press, L	1	3		
		C19 KB OH Bwd Lun. L	1	3		

#039 - Rehab

M	R	Exercise	Sets	Reps	Rest	Note
SEQUENCE	3	F01 Hurdles	1 ea.	10 ea.		Slow to moderate pace; Don't rush. Move about between rounds.
		C01 **Calf Raise**	1	10		
		C06 **Prisoner Squat**	1	10		
		F03 Down Dog / Up Dog	1	10	20s/ set, +2min/ round	
		B02 Superman Row	1	10		
		A06 Push-Up	1	10		
		E06 Bird Dog Plank	1	10		
		C18 **Lunge Walk**	1	10		

WEEK 14

#040 ☆ TEST, The BW500

M	R	Exercise	Sets	Reps	Rest	Note
		B08 Inverted Row	As req.	25		
		D12 Burpee	As req.	50		
		A06 Push-Up	As req.	50		
		C03 Air Squat	As req.	100	As req.	AQAP
		E08 Everest Mtn. Climber	As req.	100		For
		F06 Glute Bridge	As req.	100		total time
		E14 Rower Sit-Up	As req.	50		
		B08 Inverted Row	As req.	25		

#041 ☆ KB Complex No. 4

M	R	Exercise	Sets	Reps	Rest	Note
SEQUENCE	12	B05 KB Supported Row, R	1	5	None/ set, 1min/ round	
		F18 KB Clean & Press, R	1	5		
		C09 KB Front Squat, R	1	5		
		F14 KB 1h Swing, R	1	5		
		B05 KB Supported Row, L	1	5		
		F18 KB Clean & Press, L	1	5		
		C09 KB Front Squat, L	1	5		
		F14 KB 1h Swing, L	1	10		

#042 – BW Short Cycle

M	R	Exercise	Sets	Reps	Rest	Note
CIRC.	19	A17 Seated Dips	1	$1a_110d_11$	Brief/ set, 20-60s/ round	Pyramid: Ascending sets, then descending
		F04 Bird Dog	1	$2a_220d_22$		
		E13 Bicycle Crunch	1	$2a_220d_22$		
		C05 Hindu Squat	1	$2a_220d_22$		

WEEK 15

#043 ☆ BW/ Run Sequence

M	R	Exercise	Sets	Reps	Rest	Note
		ᴮ⁰⁹ **Dead Hang Low**	3	ALAP	1min	
SEQ.	8	ᴬ⁰⁶ Push-Up	1	4	None/ set, 20s/ round	
		ᶠ⁰³ Down Dog / Up Dog	1	4		
		ᴱ¹⁵ Sit-Up	1	6		
		ᶜ¹² Sk8 Squat	1	6		
		ᴳ¹⁵ Run	6	~100m	= walk	

#044 ☆ KB Complex No. 5

M	R	Exercise	Sets	Reps	Rest	Note
SEQ.	12 to 15	ᶠ¹⁸ KB Clean & Press, R	1	5	None/ set, 1min/ round	
		ᶜ⁰⁹ KB Front Squat, R	1	5		
		ᶠ¹⁴ KB 1h Swing, R	1	5		
		ᶠ¹² KB SL Deadlift, R	1	5		
		ᶠ¹⁸ KB Clean & Press, L	1	5		
		ᶜ⁰⁹ KB Front Squat, L	1	5		
		ᶠ¹⁴ KB 1h Swing, L	1	5		
		ᶠ¹² KB SL Deadlift, L	1	5		

#045 – Prof. Tabata's Curse

M	R	Exercise	Sets	Reps	Rest	Note
		ᴬ¹⁷ Seated Dips	8	20s	10s/ set, +2min/ exercise	
		ᴱ⁰⁷ **Mtn. Climber**	8	20s		
		ᴮ⁰⁵ KB Supported Row	8	20s		Fast; Alt./ set
		ᶜ⁰⁴ **Squat Jump**	8	20s		

WEEK 16

#046 ☆ The Ministry of Funny Walks

M	R	Exercise	Sets	Reps	Rest	Note
SEQUENCE	4	G01 Model Walk	1	15-20m each	15-20s/ set, +1 min/ round	
		C18 Lunge Walk	1			
		G02 Chaplin Walk	1			
		G05 Bear Walk	1			
		D09 Hzt Frog Jump	1			
		G04 Crab Walk	1			
		D11 Sprunglauf	1			
		G06 Wheelbarrow	1			

#047 ☆

M	R	Exercise	Sets	Reps	Rest	Note
		B13 **Pull-Up**	5	3	1min	Mod. as req.
CIRC.	5	E01 **High Plank**	1	40s each	none/set +1min/ round	
		C16 Static Lunge, L	1			
		C16 Static Lunge, R	1			
CIRC.	5	A06 Push-Up	1	30s each	30s/set +1min/ round	
		F19 **Windmill**	1			Alt. ea.
		F09 **Band Deadlift**	1			Heavy
		F18 KB Clean & Press	1			Light
		A16 **KB Halo**	1			Alt. ea.

#048

M	R	Exercise	Sets	Reps	Rest	Note
CIRC.	10	D02 Shuffle Jump	1	30s/ set	30s/ set	
		D04 Kick-Back Jump	1			
		F16 **KB High Swing**	1			
SEQ.	1	E01 High Plank	1	45s/ set	n/a	
		E03 Low Plank	1		n/a	
		E02 Plank	1		1min	
		E04 Side Plank	1 ea	1min ea		

WEEK 17

#049 ☆

M	R	Exercise	Sets	Reps	Rest	Note
CIRCUIT	6	B03 Seated Band Row	1	20s each set	15s/ set, +1min/ round	
		D12 Burpee	1			
		A06 Push-Up	1			
		C06 Prisoner Squat	1			
		E08 Everest Mtn. Climber	1			
		F08 SL Glute Bridge	1 ea.			
		E17 Russian Twist	1			

#050 ☆

M	R	Exercise	Sets	Reps	Rest	Note
CIRCUIT	3	B10 **Dead Hang High**	1	20s each	20s/set +1min/ round	
		B09 Dead Hang Low	1			
		B04 Standing Band Row	1			
		F11 **KB Deadlift**	1			2KB; Medium
		F13 KB 2h Swing	1			Medium
		B06 **KB Renegade Row**	1			Medium
		F17 KB Clean	1			Medium
		F07 **Elev. Glute Bridge**	1			
		E22 **Inverted Ab Tuck**	1			
		C04 Squat Jump	8	20s	10s	Tabata

#051

M	R	Exercise	Sets	Reps	Rest	Note
		E25 **KB Turkish Sit-Up**	6 ea.	3 ea.	Brief	Alt./ set
SEQ	4	F18 KB Clean & Press, R	3	1, 2, 3	Brief	Go heavy.
		F18 KB Clean & Press, L	3	1, 2, 3	Brief	Alt. ea. set.
		B13 Pull-Up	3	1, 2, 3	Brief	Don't rush.
		G14 Run-In-Place	8	20s	10s	Tabata
		C17 Bwd Lunge	4 ea.	20s	10s	KB optional

WEEK 18

#052 ☆ The Ministry of Funny Walks

M	R	Exercise	Sets	Reps	Rest	Note
SEQUENCE	3	G01 Model Walk	1	15-20m each	15-20s/ set, +1 min/ round	
		G03 **Rooster Walk**	1			
		C18 Lunge Walk	1			
		G02 Chaplin Walk	1			
		G05 Bear Walk	1			
		D09 Hzt Frog Jump	1			
		G04 Crab Walk	1			
		D11 Sprunglauf	1			
		G06 Wheelbarrow	1			
CIRC.	2	A17 Seated Dips	1	20s/ set	10s/ set, +2min after 2nd rd.	
		B08 Inverted Row	1			
		E19 Seated Leg Raise	1			
		C04 Squat Jump	1			

#053 ☆

M	R	Exercise	Sets	Reps	Rest	Note
CIRC.	5	B05 KB Supported Row	1 ea.	30s each	30s/set +1min/ round	Medium
		F09 Band Deadlift	2			Medium
		E12 Unicycle Crunch	1 ea.			
		F18 KB Clean & Press	1 ea.			Medium
		A06 Push-Up	1	AMRAP	30s	
		E03 Low Plank	1	ALAP		

#054

M	R	Exercise	Sets	Reps	Rest	Note
		E25 KB Turkish Sit-Up	5 ea.	3 ea.	Brief	Alt./ set
SEQ	5	F18 KB Clean & Press, R	3 ea.	1, 2, 3 ea.	Brief	Go heavy. Don't rush.
		F18 KB Clean & Press, L			Brief	
		B13 Pull-Up			Brief	
		G14 Run-In-Place	8	20s	10s	Tabata
		C17 Bwd Lunge	4 ea.	20s	10s	KB optional

WEEK 19

#055 ☆ BW & Run

M	R	Exercise	Sets	Reps	Rest	Note
		G15 Run	4	~100m	= walk	
SEQ.	6	A06 Push-Up	1	5	None/	
		F03 Down Dog / Up Dog	1	5	set,	
		E15 Sit-Up	1	5	20s/	
		C12 Sk8 Squat	1	5	round	
		G15 Run	4	~100m	= walk	

#056 ☆

M	R	Exercise	Sets	Reps	Rest	Note
		B13 Pull-Up	6	30-50%	45s	Mod. as req.
		A05 Incline Push-Up	1	AMRAP	2 min	
		D12 Burpee	8	20s	10s	Tabata
SS	5	C14 Step-Up, L	1	30s	n/a	
		C14 Step-Up, R	1	30s	30s	
		F19 Windmill	1	20	30s	Slow
SEQ.	3	**A13 KB Floor Press**	1 ea	5 ea	15s ea	
		F17 KB Clean	1 ea	5 ea	15s ea	1KB; Heavy
		A14 KB Press	1 ea	3 ea	15s ea	
		D07 Tuck Jump	3	10	30s	

#057

M	R	Exercise	Sets	Reps	Rest	Note
SS	15	D02 Shuffle Jump	1	30s/	30s/	
		F16 KB High Swing	1	set	set	

WEEK 20

#058 ☆ The Ministry of Funny Walks

M	R	Exercise	Sets	Reps	Rest	Note
SEQUENCE	4	G01 Model Walk	1	15-20m each	15-20s/ set, +1 min/ round	
		G03 Rooster Walk	1			
		C18 Lunge Walk	1			
		G02 Chaplin Walk	1			
		G05 Bear Walk	1			
		D09 Hzt Frog Jump	1			
		G04 Crab Walk	1			
		D11 Sprunglauf	1			
		G06 Wheelbarrow	1			
		G16 **Medicine Ball Toss**	n/a	10min	As req.	

#059 ☆

M	R	Exercise	Sets	Reps	Rest	Note
SS	3	B10 Dead Hang High	1	ALAP	1 min	
		A06 Push-Up	1	AMRAP	1 min	
SS	4	F14 KB 1h Swing, L	1	30s	30s	Medium
		F14 KB 1h Swing, R	1	30s	30s	
		C03 Air Squat	8	20s	10s	Tabata
SS	5	E24 **KB Floor Wiper**	1	10	30s	2KB
		C08 **KB H2H Sumo Sq.**	1	30	30s	Fast
		G12 **Buddy Pull**	3	15m	As req.	

#060 – BW & Run

M	R	Exercise	Sets	Reps	Rest	Note
SEQ.	10	A06 Push-Up	1	4	None/ set, 20s/ round	
		F03 Down Dog / Up Dog	1	6		
		E16 Sit-Up Twist	1	8		
		C12 Sk8 Squat	1	10		
		G15 Run	5	~100m	= walk	

WEEK 21

#061 ☆

M	R	Exercise	Sets	Reps	Rest	Note
SS	2	B11 **Negative Pull-Up**	1	AMRAP	1 min	Slowly down
		A06 Push-Up	1	AMRAP	1 min	Slowly down
		G10 **KB Pick-Up Walk**	5	30s	30s	2KB; Medium
SS	5	E12 Unicycle Crunch, L	1	20s	n/a	
		E12 Unicycle Crunch, R	1	20s	20s	
SS	3	C06 Prisoner Squat	1	5	n/a	10-count
		D06 **Vertical Jump**	1	3	30s	Max

#062 ☆

M	R	Exercise	Sets	Reps	Rest	Note
		B13 Pull-Up	10	30-50%	45s	Mod. as req.
		A06 Push-Up	As req.	5 min	2 min	AMRAP
		F11 KB Deadlift	5	10	30s	2KB; Medium
CIRC.	3	C04 Squat Jump	1	15	Brief	
		B03 Seated Band Row	1	10		
		E20 **Flat Leg Raise**	1	10		

#063 – Fibonacci's B-Sequence

M	R	Exercise	Sets	Reps	Rest	Note
SEQUENCE	1	D14 **Bastard Burpee**	2	1	10s ea.	
		D14 Bastard Burpee	1	2	10s	
		D14 Bastard Burpee	1	3	10s	
		D14 Bastard Burpee	1	5	10s	
		D13 **Push-Up Burpee**	1	8	20s	
		D13 Push-Up Burpee	1	13	20s	
		D12 Burpee	1	21	30s	
		D04 Kick-Back Jump	1	34	90s	
		B12 **Chin-Up**	As req.	30	As req.	Mod. as req.
		E-16 Sit-Up Twist	As req.	60	As req.	

WEEK 22

#064 ☆

M	R	Exercise	Sets	Reps	Rest	Note
CIRCUIT	5	B08 Inverted Row	1			
		F17 KB Clean	1			
		F13 KB 2h Swing	1	20s each	20s/set +1min/ round	Medium
		F12 KB SL Deadlift, L	1			
		F12 KB SL Deadlift, R	1			
		C07 KB Goblet Squat	1			
		E05 **X-Kick High Plank**	4	1 min	30s	
		E07 Mtn. Climber	8	20s	10s	Tabata

#065 ☆

M	R	Exercise	Sets	Reps	Rest	Note
SS	5	B07 KB High Pull, R	1	12	n/a	
		B07 KB High Pull, L	1	12	30s	
		A06 Push-Up	AMAP	$1a_1$Max	S/U	Until failure
		C03 Air Squat	8	20s	10s	Tabata
		E11 Reverse Crunch	1	30	30s	
		F19 Windmill	1	20	30s	Slow; Alt. ea.
		A15 **KB OH Static**	3	1min	1min	2KB
		G11 **Buddy Carry**	3	30m	1min	

#066 - BW & Run

M	R	Exercise	Sets	Reps	Rest	Note
SEQ.	10	E19 Seated Leg Raise	1	6	None/ set, 30s/ round	
		A17 Seated Dips	1	6		
		F03 Down Dog / Up Dog	1	6		
		C12 Sk8 Squat	1	6		
		G15 Run	6	~100m	= walk	

WEEK 23

#067 ☆

M	R	Exercise	Sets	Reps	Rest	Note
		B13 Pull-Up	10	30-50%	45s	Mod. as req.
CIRCUIT	5	F10 **KB Sumo Deadlift**	1	30s each	30s/set +1min/ round	Heavy
		A13 KB Floor Press	1			2KB
		B06 KB Renegade Row	1			2KB
		E18 **KB Russian Twist**	1			
		D08 **Box Jump**	Minim.	40	Minim.	AQAP
		G12 Buddy Pull	3	30m	1min	

#068 ☆

M	R	Exercise	Sets	Reps	Rest	Note
		B13 Pull-Up	1	AMRAP	1min	Mod. as req.
		A06 Push-Up	2	AMRAP	1min	10-count
CIRCUIT	3	F13 KB 2h Swing	1	20s each	20s/set +1min/ round	Medium
		C14 Step-Up, L	1			
		C14 Step-Up, R	1			
		E21 **Hanging Leg Raise**	1			
		F21 **KB Windmill**, L	1			Light
		F21 KB Windmill, R	1			Light
		D13 Push-Up Burpee	n/a	25	n/a	AQAP

#069 – The Ministry of Funny Walks

M	R	Exercise	Sets	Reps	Rest	Note
SEQUENCE	4	G01 Model Walk	1	15-20m each	15-20s/ set, +1 min/ round	
		G03 Rooster Walk	1			
		C18 Lunge Walk	1			
		G02 Chaplin Walk	1			
		G05 Bear Walk	1			
		D09 Hzt Frog Jump	1			
		G04 Crab Walk	1			
		D11 Sprunglauf	1			
		G06 Wheelbarrow	1			

WEEK 24

#070 ☆

M	R	Exercise	Sets	Reps	Rest	Note
SS	5	B08 Inverted Row	1	10	30s	
		A12 **Walking Push-Up**	1	10	30s	
CIRC.	2	C15 Step-Up Jump	1	30s each	20s/set	
		F15 **KB H2H Swing**	1			
		F21 KB Windmill	1			
SEQ.	3	G09 **KB Waiter Walk**	1	20s each	1min/ round	2KB
		G08 **KB Rack Walk**	1			
		G07 **KB Farmer Walk**	1			

#071 ☆

M	R	Exercise	Sets	Reps	Rest	Note
		B13 Pull-Up	10	30-50%	45s	Mod. as req.
SEQ.	5	F13 KB 2h Swing	1	20s each	1min/ round	
		F14 KB 1h Swing, R	1			
		F14 KB 1h Swing, L	1			
		F15 KB H2H Swing	1			
		A06 Push-Up	1	AMRAP	1min	
		E07 Mtn. Climber	8	20s	10s	Tabata
		D12 Burpee	8	20s	10s	Tabata

#072

M	R	Exercise	Sets	Reps	Rest	Note
SS	15	D02 Shuffle Jump	1	30s/ set	30s/ set	
		F16 KB High Swing	1			
		G16 Medicine Ball Toss	n/a	5min	As req.	

WEEK 25

#073 ☆ TEST, The BW500

M	R	Exercise	Sets	Reps	Rest	Note
		B08 Inverted Row	As req.	25	As req.	AQAP For total time
		D12 Burpee	As req.	50		
		A06 Push-Up	As req.	50		
		C03 Air Squat	As req.	100		
		E08 Everest Mtn. Climber	As req.	100		
		F06 Glute Bridge	As req.	100		
		E14 Rower Sit-Up	As req.	50		
		B08 Inverted Row	As req.	25		

#074 ☆

M	R	Exercise	Sets	Reps	Rest	Note
		B06 KB Renegade Row	3	10	30s	Alt. ea.
		F11 KB Deadlift	1	25	1min	2KB
		E01 High Plank	1	ALAP	1min	
		A15 KB OH Static	2	ALAP	1min	
CIRC.	5	**C13 Bulgarian Split Sq., L**	1	20s each	10s/set +30s/ round	1KB@chest
		C13 Bulgarian Split Sq., R	1			1KB@chest
		B04 Standing Band Row	1			

#075 - BW & Run

M	R	Exercise	Sets	Reps	Rest	Note
SEQ.	12	A06 Push-Up	1	6	None/ set, 30s/ round	
		F03 Down Dog / Up Dog	1	6		
		E15 Sit-Up	1	6		
		C12 Sk8 Squat	1	6		
		G15 Run	6	~100m	= walk	

WEEK 26

#076 ☆

M	R	Exercise	Sets	Reps	Rest	Note
CIRC.	2	B03 Seated Band Row	2	20s/ set	10s/set, +1min/ round	
		B01 Bat Wings	2			
		F11 KB Deadlift	2			2KB; Medium
		F08 SL Glute Bridge	1 ea.			
		A06 Push-Up	1	25	n/a	
		D10 Lunge Jump	2	8	30s	
SS	5	E18 KB Russian Twist	1	30s	30s	Light
		A16 KB Halo	1	30s	30s	Alt. ea.
SS	3	**C10 KB OH Squat**, R	1	8	30s	
		C10 KB OH Squat, L	1	8	30s	

#077 ☆

M	R	Exercise	Sets	Reps	Rest	Note
		B11 Negative Pull-Up	1	AMRAP	1min	
		F13 KB 2h Swing	1	30	1min	Light
		A08 Diamond Push-Up	1	AMRAP	1min	
		D08 Box Jump	1	25	1min	Go high
		E20 Flat Leg Raise	1	20	1min	
SS	5	F17 KB Clean, R	1	15	30s	
		F17 KB Clean, L	1	15	30s	
		D03 Zig Zag Jump	3	30s	30s	

#078

M	R	Exercise	Sets	Reps	Rest	Note
		B08 Inverted Row	2	15	30s	
SS	3	F15 KB H2H Swing	1	15	30s	Medium
		C07 KB Goblet Squat	1	15	30s	
		E08 Everest Mtn. Climber	1	30	1min	Light
		E24 KB Floor Wiper	1	20	1min	2KB
		C10 KB OH Squat, R	1	15	30s	
		C10 KB OH Squat, L	1	15	1min	
		G11 Buddy Carry	3	20m	1min	

WEEK 27

#079 ☆

M	R	Exercise	Sets	Reps	Rest	Note
		B10 Dead Hang High	1	ALAP	1min	
		F11 KB Deadlift	3	4	2min	2KB; X-Heavy
CIRCUIT	4	F03 Down Dog / Up Dog	1	30s each	15s/set +1min/ round	
		C13 Bulgarian Split Sq., R	1			KB optional
		C13 Bulgarian Split Sq., L	1			KB optional
		E12 Unicycle Crunch, R	1			
		E12 Unicycle Crunch, L	1			
		E03 Low Plank	1			

#080 ☆

M	R	Exercise	Sets	Reps	Rest	Note
		B13 Pull-Up	1	AMRAP	3min	Mod. as req.
		B10 Dead Hang High	1	ALAP	2min	
		B09 Dead Hang Low	1	ALAP	1min	
		F11 KB Deadlift	1	30	1min	2KB; Light
CIRC.	5	F17 KB Clean	1	30s each	20s/set +1min/ round	Alt. ea.; Fast
		C04 Squat Jump	1			Light
		E18 KB Russian Twist	1			
		B03 Seated Band Row	1			Heavy

#081 ☆

M	R	Exercise	Sets	Reps	Rest	Note
		B08 Inverted Row	1	10	1min	
		F11 KB Deadlift	1	50	As req.	2KB; Medium
		A06 Push-Up	1	50%	1min	
		D10 Lunge Jump	2	10	30s	
SEQ.	3	E02 Plank	1	40s each	1min after round	
		F04 Bird Dog	1			
		E05 X-Kick High Plank	1			
SS	4	A14 KB Press	1 ea.	10 ea.	30s	
		E07 Mtn. Climber	1	40	30s	

WEEK 28

#082 ☆

M	R	Exercise	Sets	Reps	Rest	Note
		^{B06} KB Renegade Row	1	10	1min	
SEQ.	3	^{F13} KB 2h Swing	1	20s each	40s after each round	Medium
		^{F14} KB 1h Swing, R	1			
		^{F14} KB 1h Swing, L	1			
		^{F15} KB H2H Swing	1			
SS	3	^{A07} **Decline Push-Up**	1	10	n/a	
		^{E20} Flat Leg Raise	1	10	1min	
		^{F17} KB Clean	5 ea.	5 ea.	1min	Heavy
		^{D01} Jumping Jack	3	1min	30s	

#083 ☆

M	R	Exercise	Sets	Reps	Rest	Note
		^{B13} Pull-Up	3	AMRAP	1min	Mod. as req.
		^{F14} KB 1h Swing	5 ea.	30s ea.	30s	Light
		^{D08} Box Jump	n/a	50	As req.	1st set 15-20
		^{A14} KB Press	4 ea.	30s ea.	30s ea.	Light; Slow
SEQ.	3	^{G07} KB Farmer Walk	1 ea.	20s each	1min after full round	1 KB Medium
		^{G08} KB Rack Walk	1 ea.			
		^{G09} KB Waiter Walk	1 ea.			

#084 ☆

M	R	Exercise	Sets	Reps	Rest	Note
SS	3	^{B04} Standing Band Row	3	15	n/a	Heavy
		^{A11} **Band Push-Up**	3	10	1min	
		^{F11} KB Deadlift	10	4	45s	2KB; Heavy
		^{C06} Prisoner Squat	1	25	30s	Slow
		^{F21} KB Windmill	2 ea.	5 ea.	30s	Medium
		^{E18} KB Russian Twist	2	20	30s	

WEEK 29

#085 ☆

M	R	Exercise	Sets	Reps	Rest	Note
		E26 **KB Turkish Half-Up**	n/a	8 ea.	Brief	Alt. ea.
CIRCUIT	4	B13 Pull-Up	1	10	20s/set +2min/ round	Mod. as req.
		F10 KB Sumo Deadlift	1	10		Heavy
		A06 Push-Up	1	10		
		D08 Box Jump	1	10		
		F18 KB Clean & Press	1	10 ea.		Medium

#086 ☆

M	R	Exercise	Sets	Reps	Rest	Note
SS	5	B13 Pull-Up	1	5	30s	Mod. as req.
		F11 KB Deadlift	1	10	30s	2KB; Med.
SS	5	A07 Decline Push-Up	1	10	Brief	
		C16 Static Lunge	1 ea.	45s ea.	30s, 2nd	
SS	5	E16 Sit-Up Twist	1	10	Brief	
		C10 KB OH Squat	1 ea.	10 ea.	30s, 2nd	Medium
		G12 Buddy Pull	3	30m	1min	Medium; Fast

#087

M	R	Exercise	Sets	Reps	Rest	Note
		B06 KB Renegade Row	1	10	1min	
SEQ.	3	F13 KB 2h Swing	1	30s each	1min after each round	Medium
		F14 KB 1h Swing, R	1			
		F14 KB 1h Swing, L	1			
		F15 KB H2H Swing	1			
		A12 Walking Push-Up	5	30s	30s	
SS	3	E12 Unicycle Crunch	1 ea.	15 ea.	30s, 2nd	
		F21 KB Windmill	1 ea.	10 ea.	30s, 2nd	Medium
		D07 Tuck Jump	3	30s	15s	Heavy
		G13 **Reverse Buddy Pull**	5	20m	1min	

WEEK 30

#088 ☆

M	R	Exercise	Sets	Reps	Rest	Note
		^{E26} KB Turkish Half-Up	n/a	10 ea.	Brief	Alt ea.
		^{B11} Negative Pull-Up	1	AMRAP	1min	Mod. as req.
		^{F11} KB Deadlift	5	5	1min	2KB;X-Heavy
		^{A06} Push-Up	10	10	30s ea.	Stop@failure
		^{D10} Lunge Jump	8	20s	10s	Tabata
		^{E23} **Ab Roll-Out**	3	AMRAP	1min	

#089 ☆

M	R	Exercise	Sets	Reps	Rest	Note
		^{B08} Inverted Row	1	10	1min	
		^{F09} Band Deadlift	3	10	20s	
		^{A09} **Wide Push-Up**	1	AMRAP	1min	
		^{E24} KB Floor Wiper	5	10	30s	2KB; Med.
		^{G15} Run	4	50m	= Walk	80%
		^{E12} Unicycle Crunch	6 ea.	20s ea.	10s ea.	Alt. sets

#090 – Circuit No. 4

M	R	Exercise	Sets	Reps	Rest	Note
CIRCUIT	4	^{B13} Pull-Up	1	20s/ set	20s/set +2min/ round	Mod. as req.
		^{G10} KB Pick-Up Walk	1			2KB; Heavy
		^{A06} Push-Up	1			
		^{E24} KB Floor Wiper	1			2KB; Med.
		^{D08} Box Jump	1			
		^{F18} KB Clean & Press	1			Alt. ea.; Med.

WEEK 31

#091 ☆

M	R	Exercise	Sets	Reps	Rest	Note
CIRC.	10	B13 Pull-Up	1	4	20s/set	Mod. as req.
		F11 KB Deadlift	1	4		2KB
		E20 Flat Leg Raise	1	8		
CIRCUIT	3	D07 Tuck Jump	1	15s each	15s/set +1min/ round	Fast
		A10 Plyo Push-Up	1			
		E18 KB Russian Twist	1			Fast
		A14 KB Press, R	1			Light; Fast
		A14 KB Press, L	1			Light; Fast

#092 ☆

M	R	Exercise	Sets	Reps	Rest	Note
		A06 Push-Up	10	$10d_11$	S-Up	Descend 1 ea.
		C20 KB Lunge Walk	3	30s	30s	2KB; Medium
		E25 KB Turkish Sit-Up	2 ea.	30s ea.	30s ea.	Medium
		F17 KB Clean	3 ea.	10 ea.	30s ea.	Heavy; Alt.set
		G16 Medicine Ball Toss	n/a	5min	As req.	

#093

M	R	Exercise	Sets	Reps	Rest	Note
		B08 Inverted Row	3	10	30s	
CIRCUIT	4	F13 KB 2h Swing	1	30s each	20s/set +1min/ round	2KB; Medium
		D08 Box Jump	1			2KB; Medium
		F18 KB Clean & Press, L	1			Heavy; Alt.set
		F18 KB Clean & Press, R	1			
		E23 Ab Roll-Out	3	AMRAP	30s	

WEEK 32

#094

M	R	Exercise	Sets	Reps	Rest	Note
CIRCUIT	3	B06 KB Renegade Row	2	30s each	20s/set +1min/ round	Medium
		F12 KB SL Deadlift	1 ea.			2KB; Medium
		D05 Vertical Frog Jump	2			
		A17 Seated Dips	2			Heavy; Alt.set
		E12 Unicycle Crunch	1 ea.			
		G12 Buddy Pull	3	30m	1min	

#095

M	R	Exercise	Sets	Reps	Rest	Note
		A06 Push-Up	10	$1a_1 10$	S-Up	Ascend 1 ea.
CIRCUIT	3	C07 KB Goblet Squat	2	20s each	20s/set +1min/ round	
		E25 KB Turkish Sit-Up	1 ea.			2KB; Medium
		A14 KB Press	1 ea.			Med.; Alt. sets
		F17 KB Clean	1 ea.			Alt. ea.
		G16 Medicine Ball Toss	n/a	10min	As req.	

#096

M	R	Exercise	Sets	Reps	Rest	Note
SS	10	B13 Pull-Up	1	5	30s	Mod. as req.
		F11 KB Deadlift	1	5	30s	2KB; Heavy
CIRCUIT	2	A13 KB Floor Press	2	30s each	20s/set +1min/ round	2 KB; Med.
		C13 Bulgarian Split Sq.	1 ea.			KB optional
		F20 KB Low Windmill	1 ea.			Heavy
		F17 KB Clean	2			Med.; Alt. ea.
		D12 Burpee	2			
		G12 Buddy Pull	5	20m	1min	

WEEK 33

#097 ☆

M	R	Exercise	Sets	Reps	Rest	Note
CIRCUIT	1	B10 Dead Hang High	1	ALAP	1min	
		F11 KB Deadlift	5	5	30s	2KB; Heavy
		D08 Box Jump	5	10	30s	2KB; Medium
		F17 KB Clean	5 ea.	10 ea.	30s ea.	Med.; Alt.set
		F22 **Sledgehammer**	5	30s	30s	

#098 ☆

M	R	Exercise	Sets	Reps	Rest	Note
		B07 KB High Pull	3 ea.	30s ea.	30s ea.	Medium
		F13 KB 2h Swing	1	1min	1min	Light
		A12 Walking Push-Up	3	30s	30s	
		E10 Static Crunch	1	1min	1min	
		C11 **KB Thruster**	4	15	30s	2KB; Light

#099

M	R	Exercise	Sets	Reps	Rest	Note
SS	10	B13 Pull-Up	1	5	30s	Mod. as req.
		F11 KB Deadlift	1	5	30s	2KB; Medium
CIRCUIT	6	A11 Band Push-Up	1	20s each	15s/set +30s/ round	
		D07 Tuck Jump	1			
		A17 Seated Dips	1			
		E22 Inverted Ab Tuck	1			

WEEK 34

#100 ☆

M	R	Exercise	Sets	Reps	Rest	Note
		^{A06} Push-Up	11	11d$_1$1	S-Up	Descend 1 ea.
CIRC.	3	^{C20} KB Lunge Walk	1	30s/ set	30s/ set, 1min/ round	2KB
		^{E24} KB Floor Wiper	1			2KB
		^{F17} KB Clean	1			2KB
		^{D12} Burpee	1			
		^{G12} Buddy Pull	4	30m	1min	

#101 ☆

M	R	Exercise	Sets	Reps	Rest	Note
		^{B08} Inverted Row	2	15	45s	.
		^{F13} KB 2h Swing	4	45s	15s	Light/Med.
		^{D08} Box Jump	4	12	30s	
		^{F18} KB Clean & Press	4	30s	30s	Alt. ea.; Fast
		^{E08} Everest Mtn. Climber	4	30s	30s	
		^{G13} Reverse Buddy Pull	4	20m	1min	

#102

M	R	Exercise	Sets	Reps	Rest	Note
		^{B06} KB Renegade Row	1	40s each	20s/set +1min/ round	2KB; Alt. ea.
CIRCUIT	5	^{F12} KB SL Deadlift, L	1			
		^{F12} KB SL Deadlift, R	1			
		^{A08} Diamond Push-Up	1			
		^{D12} Burpee	1			
		^{D10} Lunge Jump	1			Alt. ea.

WEEK 35

#103 ☆ TEST, The BW500

M	R	Exercise	Sets	Reps	Rest	Note
		^{B08} Inverted Row	As req.	25		
		^{D12} Burpee	As req.	50		
		^{A06} Push-Up	As req.	50		AQAP
		^{C03} Air Squat	As req.	100	As req.	
		^{E08} Everest Mtn. Climber	As req.	100		For
		^{F06} Glute Bridge	As req.	100		total time
		^{E14} Rower Sit-Up	As req.	50		
		^{B08} Inverted Row	As req.	25		

#104 ☆ Circuit No. 2

M	R	Exercise	Sets	Reps	Rest	Note
CIRCUIT	2	^{F12} KB SL Deadlift	1 ea.	30s each set	15s/ set, +2min/ round	
		^{C07} KB Goblet Squat	2			
		^{F18} KB Clean & Press	1 ea.			
		^{F14} KB 1h Swing	1 ea.			
		^{B05} KB Supported Row	1 ea.			
		^{C17} Bwd Lunge	1 ea.			
		^{F04} Bird Dog	1 ea.			
		^{F02} Dirty Dog	1 ea.			
		^{D03} Zig Zag Jump	2			
		^{A01} Band Push	2			
		^{E12} Unicycle Crunch	1 ea.			

#105 – Circuit No. 4

M	R	Exercise	Sets	Reps	Rest	Note
CIRCUIT	5	^{B13} Pull-Up	1	10	20s/set +2min/ round	Mod. as req.
		^{F11} KB Deadlift	1	10		2KB; Heavy
		^{A11} Band Push-Up	1	10		
		^{E24} KB Floor Wiper	1	10		2KB; Medium
		^{D08} Box Jump	1	10		
		^{F18} KB Clean & Press	1	5 ea.		Medium

WEEK 36

#106 ☆

M	R	Exercise	Sets	Reps	Rest	Note
SS	12	B13 Pull-Up	1	5	30s	Mod. as req.
		F11 KB Deadlift	1	5	30s	2KB; Heavy
CIRCUIT	2	A09 Wide Push-Up	2	30s each	20s/set +1min/ round	
		C13 Bulgarian Split Sq.	1 ea.			KB optional
		F20 KB Low Windmill	1 ea.			Heavy
		F17 KB Clean	2			Med.; Alt. ea.
		B03 Seated Band Row	2			
		G07 KB Farmer Walk	3	30m	1min	

#107 ☆

M	R	Exercise	Sets	Reps	Rest	Note
		A06 Push-Up	11	$1a_1 11$	n/a	Descend 1 ea.
		C14 Step-Up	2 ea.	10 ea.	30s, 2nd	
		E26 KB Turkish Half-Up	3 ea.	6 ea.	30s ea.	Medium
		F21 KB Windmill	3 ea.	5 ea.	30s, 2nd	Medium
		E07 Mtn. Climber	8	20s	10s/ set, 1min/ exercise	Tabata. Alt. sets on KBs
		F17 KB Clean	8	20s		
		B07 KB High Pull	8	20s		

#108

M	R	Exercise	Sets	Reps	Rest	Note
SS	15	E22 Inverted Ab Tuck	1	6	n/a	
		F16 KB High Swing	1	12	1min	

WEEK 37

#109 ☆

M	R	Exercise	Sets	Reps	Rest	Note
		E27 **KB Turkish Get-Up**	n/a	15min	As req.	Focus on form
		B10 Dead Hang High	1	ALAP	1min	.
		F10 KB Sumo Deadlift	5	8	1min	Heavy
		D08 Box Jump	5	15	20s	
		F18 KB Clean & Press	4 ea.	15 ea.	30s ea.	Alt. sets
		D13 Push-Up Burpee	4	30s	30s	
		G12 Buddy Pull	4	30m	1min	

#110 ☆

M	R	Exercise	Sets	Reps	Rest	Note
CIRCUIT	3	B07 KB High Pull	1 ea.	20s ea.	20s/set +2min/ round	Medium
		F13 KB 2h Swing	1	40s		Medium
		C07 KB Goblet Squat	1	40s		Medium
		F19 Windmill	1	40s		Alt. ea.
		A12 Walking Push-Up	1	40s		
		E11 Reverse Crunch	1	40s		No load

#111 – The Ministry of Funny Walks

M	R	Exercise	Sets	Reps	Rest	Note
SEQUENCE	4	G01 Model Walk	1	15-20m each	15-20s/ set, +1 min/ round	
		G03 Rooster Walk	1			
		C18 Lunge Walk	1			
		G02 Chaplin Walk	1			
		G05 Bear Walk	1			
		D09 Hzt Frog Jump	1			
		G04 Crab Walk	1			
		D11 Sprunglauf	1			
		G06 Wheelbarrow	1			

WEEK 38

#112 ☆ The Brief Abduction of Fran

M	R	Exercise	Sets	Reps	Rest	Note
SEQUENCE	2	B13 Pull-Up	1	9	Brief, +5min after round	Each round AQAP
		C11 KB Thruster, 2KB	1	9		
		B13 Pull-Up	1	6		
		C11 KB Thruster, 2KB	1	6		
		B13 Pull-Up	1	3		
		C11 KB Thruster, 2KB	1	3		

#113 ☆

M	R	Exercise	Sets	Reps	Rest	Note
SS	12	B12 Chin-Up	1	5	30s	Mod. as req.
		F11 KB Deadlift	1	5	30s	2KB; Heavy
CIRCUIT	4	A08 Diamond Push-Up	1	AMRAP	1min	
		C04 Squat Jump	1	20s each	20s/ set	
		B06 KB Renegade Row	1			2KB; Alt. ea.
		F17 KB Clean	1			Heavy; Alt.ea.
		C11 KB Thruster	1			2KB; Fast
		F22 Sledgehammer	1			

#114 BW & Run

M	R	Exercise	Sets	Reps	Rest	Note
SEQ.	6	A10 Plyo Push-Up	1	5	10s	
		F03 Down Dog / Up Dog	1	5	10s	
		E23 Ab Roll-Out	1	5	10s	
		D06 Vertical Jump	1	5	10s	
		G15 Run	1	~200m	90s	Walk to rest

WEEK 39

#115 ☆ Circuit No. 2

M	R	Exercise	Sets	Reps	Rest	Note
CIRCUIT	2	F12 KB SL Deadlift	1 ea.	30s each set	15s/ set, +2min/ round	
		C07 KB Goblet Squat	2			
		F18 KB Clean & Press	1 ea.			
		F14 KB 1h Swing	1 ea.			
		B05 KB Supported Row	1 ea.			
		C17 Bwd Lunge	1 ea.			
		F04 Bird Dog	1 ea.			
		F02 Dirty Dog	1 ea.			
		D03 Zig Zag Jump	2			
		A01 Band Push	2			
		E12 Unicycle Crunch	1 ea.			

#116 ☆

M	R	Exercise	Sets	Reps	Rest	Note
		A06 Push-Up	11	11d$_1$1	n/a	Descend 1 ea.
		C19 KB OH Bwd Lunge	4 ea.	30s ea.	30s ea.	Medium
		E24 KB Floor Wiper	4	15	30s	2KB
		C10 KB OH Squat	1 ea.	10 ea.	30s ea.	Medium
SEQ.	5	E05 X-Kick High Plank	1	30s each	30s/ round	
		E02 Plank	1			
		C08 KB H2H Sumo Squat	1			

#117

M	R	Exercise	Sets	Reps	Rest	Note
		E27 KB Turkish Get-Up	n/a	15min	Brief	Alt ea.
SEQUENCE	3	C15 Step-Up Jump	1	20s each	10s/ set, +1min/ round	
		F13 KB 2h Swing	1			
		A03 Half Push-Up	1			Fast
		F13 KB 2h Swing	1			
		C04 Squat Jump	1			
		F13 KB 2h Swing	1			
		E09 Crunch	1			Fast
		F13 KB 2h Swing	1			

WEEK 40

#118 ☆ Fit for the Cross 1

M	R	Exercise	Sets	Reps	Rest	Note
		C18 Lunge Walk	As req.	80	As req.	In sequence, AQAP.
		E15 Sit-Up	As req.	70	As req.	
		F08 SL Glute Bridge	As req.	60	As req.	
		E20 Flat Leg Raise	As req.	50	As req.	Break up into manageable sets.
		A06 Push-Up	As req.	40	As req.	
		B08 Inverted Row	As req.	30	As req.	
		E27 KB Turkish Get-Up	n/a	10 ea.	As req.	

#119 ☆

M	R	Exercise	Sets	Reps	Rest	Note
		B11 Negative Pull-Up	5	10	1min	Mod. if req.
SEQ.	3	F13 KB 2h Swing	1	30s each	1min/ round	Medium
		F14 KB 1h Swing, R	1			
		F14 KB 1h Swing, L	1			
		F15 KB H2H Swing	1			
		D07 Tuck Jump	2	15	30s	
CIRC.	3	C11 KB Thruster	1	30s each	30s/ round	2KB
		E08 Everest Mtn. Climber	1			
		D01 Jumping Jack	1			

#120 - Rehab

M	R	Exercise	Sets	Reps	Rest	Note
SEQUENCE	6	F01 Hurdles	1 ea.	6 ea.	Brief/ set, +2min/ round	Slow to moderate pace; Don't rush. Move about between rounds.
		C01 Calf Raise	1	6		
		C06 Prisoner Squat	1	6		
		F03 Down Dog / Up Dog	1	6		
		B02 Superman Row	1	6		
		A06 Push-Up	1	6		
		E06 Bird Dog Plank	1	6		
		C18 Lunge Walk	1	6		

WEEK 41

#121 ☆ The NeverEnding Story

M	R	Exercise	Sets	Reps	Rest	Note
CIRCUIT	1	D12 Burpee	2	30s	20s/ set	
		A06 Push-Up	2			
		C06 Prisoner Squat	2			
		E08 Everest Mtn. Climber	2			
		F07 Elevated Glute Bridge	2			
		E14 Rower Sit-Up	2			
		C05 Hindu Squat	2			
		B02 Superman Row	2			
		A17 Seated Dips	2			
		C14 Step-Up	1 ea.			
		E09 Crunch	2			
		B01 Bat Wings	2			
		C02 Air Bench	2			
		F05 Straight Bridge, Static	2			
		E02 Plank	2			
		E04 Side Plank	1 ea.			
		F03 Down Dog / Up Dog	2			

#122 ☆

M	R	Exercise	Sets	Reps	Rest	Note
		B08 Inverted Row	4	15	20s	
		F12 KB SL Deadlift	4 ea.	30s ea.	30s ea.	
		A09 Wide Push-Up	5	15	20s	
		E18 KB Russian Twist	5	40s	20s	
CIRCUIT	3	B07 KB High Pull, R	1	30s each	10s/ set, +1min/ round	
		B07 KB High Pull, L	1			
		C11 KB Thruster	1			2KB
		C04 Squat Jump	1			
		A12 Walking Push-Up	1			

#123

M	R	Exercise	Sets	Reps	Rest	Note
		F16 KB High Swing	20	30s	30s	

WEEK 42

#124 ☆ Best Buddies

M	R	Exercise	Sets	Reps	Rest	Note
		G16 Medicine Ball Toss	n/a	10min	As req.	
SEQ.	3	G06 Wheelbarrow	2			
		G11 Buddy Carry	2	20m each	1min each	
		G12 Buddy Pull	2			
		G13 Reverse Buddy Pull	2			

#125 ☆

M	R	Exercise	Sets	Reps	Rest	Note
		B13 Pull-Up	n/a	25	As req.	AQAP
		F11 KB Deadlift	6	5	1min	2KB; Heavy
		A17 Seated Dips	1	1min	1min	
		C13 Bulgarian Split Sq.	3 ea.	10 ea.	30s	2KB; Alt.set
		B08 Inverted Row	5	10	30s	
		G13 Reverse Buddy Pull	4	20m	1min	

#126

M	R	Exercise	Sets	Reps	Rest	Note
		E27 KB Turkish Get-Up	n/a	15min	Brief	Alt. ea.
SEQUENCE	3	C15 Step-Up Jump	1			
		F13 KB 2h Swing	1			
		A03 Half Push-Up	1			Fast
		F13 KB 2h Swing	1	20s each	10s/ set, +1min/ round	
		C04 Squat Jump	1			
		F13 KB 2h Swing	1			
		E09 Crunch	1			Fast
		F13 KB 2h Swing	1			

WEEK 43

#127 ☆ Fibonacci's B-Sequence

M	R	Exercise	Sets	Reps	Rest	Note
SEQUENCE	1	D14 Bastard Burpee	2	1	10s ea.	
		D14 Bastard Burpee	1	2	10s	
		D14 Bastard Burpee	1	3	10s	
		D14 Bastard Burpee	1	5	10s	
		D14 Bastard Burpee	1	8	20s	
		D13 Push-Up Burpee	1	13	20s	
		D13 Push-Up Burpee	1	21	30s	
		D12 Burpee	1	34	30s	
		D04 Kick-Back Jump	1	55	5min	
		B12 Chin-Up	As req.	50	As req.	
		E-16 Sit-Up Twist	As req.	100	As req.	

#128 ☆

M	R	Exercise	Sets	Reps	Rest	Note
CIRCUIT	4	A10 Plyo Push-Up	n/a	30	As req.	AQAP
		C07 KB Goblet Squat	1	20s	30s	Heavy
		E24 KB Floor Wiper	1	20s	30s	2KB
		F18 KB Clean & Press	1	20s	30s	Alt. ea.; Heavy
		E08 Everest Mtn. Climber	1	20s	30s	

#129 – Prof. Tabata's Curse

M	R	Exercise	Sets	Reps	Rest	Note
		A17 Seated Dips	8	20s	10s/ set, +2min/ exercise	
		E07 Mtn. Climber	8	20s		
		B07 KB High Pull	8	20s		Alt./ set
		D02 Shuffle Jump	8	20s		

WEEK 44

#130 ☆ TEST, The BW500

M	R	Exercise	Sets	Reps	Rest	Note
		B08 Inverted Row	As req.	25		
		D12 Burpee	As req.	50		
		A06 Push-Up	As req.	50		AQAP
		C03 Air Squat	As req.	100	As req.	
		E08 Everest Mtn. Climber	As req.	100		For
		F06 Glute Bridge	As req.	100		total time
		E14 Rower Sit-Up	As req.	50		
		B08 Inverted Row	As req.	25		

#131 ☆

M	R	Exercise	Sets	Reps	Rest	Note
		E27 KB Turkish Get-Up	n/a	10min	As req.	
		B08 Inverted Row	1	10	1min	Hold 3s ea.
		F13 KB 2h Swing	5	10	1min	Heavy/ 2KB
		C03 Air Squat	8	20s	10s	Tabata
		D10 Lunge Jump	4	30s	30s	
		F17 KB Clean	5 ea.	5 ea.	30s ea.	Heavy
		B04 Standing Band Row	3	40s	20s	
		G07 KB Farmer Walk	3	30m	1min	Heavy

#132 - Rehab

M	R	Exercise	Sets	Reps	Rest	Note
SEQUENCE	6	F01 Hurdles	1 ea.	6 ea.	Brief/ set, +2min/ round	Slow to moderate pace; Don't rush. Move about between rounds.
		C01 Calf Raise	1	6		
		C06 Prisoner Squat	1	6		
		F03 Down Dog / Up Dog	1	6		
		B02 Superman Row	1	6		
		A06 Push-Up	1	6		
		E06 Bird Dog Plank	1	6		
		C18 Lunge Walk	1	6		

WEEK 45

#133 ☆ The NeverEnding Story 2

M	R	Exercise	Sets	Reps	Rest	Note
CIRCUIT	1	D12 Burpee	2	30s/ set	20s/ set	
		A06 Push-Up	2			
		C03 Air Squat	2			
		E08 Everest Mtn. Climber	2			
		F07 Elevated Glute Bridge	2			
		E14 Rower Sit-Up	2			
		C05 Hindu Squat	2			
		B02 Superman Row	2			
		A17 Seated Dips	2			
		C14 Step-Up	1 ea.			
		E09 Crunch	2			
		B01 Bat Wings	2			
		C17 Bwd Lunge	1 ea.			
		F04 Bird Dog	1 ea.			
		F02 Dirty Dog	1 ea.			
		D03 Zig Zag Jump	2			
		A01 Band Push	2			
		E12 Unicycle Crunch	1 ea.			
		E05 X-Kick High Plank	2			
		E04 Side Plank	1 ea.			
		F03 Down Dog / Up Dog	2			

#134 ☆ The Modified 300

M	R	Exercise	Sets	Reps	Rest	Note
		B13 Pull-Up	As req.	25	As req.	
		F11 KB Deadlift	As req.	50		2KB; Heavy
		A06 Push-Up	As req.	50		
		E24 KB Floor Wiper	As req.	50		2KB; Alt. ea.
		D08 Box Jump	As req.	50		
		F18 KB Clean & Press	As req.	50		Alt. ea.
		B13 Pull-Up	As req.	25		

#135

M	R	Exercise	Sets	Reps	Rest	Note
		G07 / G09 KB Walks	As req.	1mile	As req.	Alt. as req.

WEEK 46

#136 ☆ Circuit No. 1

M	R	Exercise	Sets	Reps	Rest	Note
CIRCUIT	2	^{C05} Hindu Squat	2	40s each set	20s/ set, +2min/ round	
		^{B02} Superman Row	2			
		^{A17} Seated Dips	2			
		^{C17} Bwd Lunge	1 ea.			Opt.: 2KB
		^{E22} Inverted Ab Tuck	2			
		^{B03} Seated Band Row	2			Hold 5s ea.
		^{C02} Air Bench	2			Optional: No rest between sets
		^{F05} Straight Bridge, Static	2			
		^{E05} X-Kick High Plank	2			
		^{E04} Side Plank	1 ea.			

#137 ☆ Swingers

M	R	Exercise	Sets	Reps	Rest	Note
		^{E27} KB Turkish Get-Up	n/a	10min	Brief	Alt. ea.
SEQUENCE	2	^{C15} Step-Up Jump	1	20s each	10s/ set, +1min/ round	
		^{F13} KB 2h Swing	1			
		^{A03} Half Push-Up	1			Fast
		^{F13} KB 2h Swing	1			
		^{C04} Squat Jump	1			
		^{F13} KB 2h Swing	1			
		^{E09} Crunch	1			Fast
		^{F13} KB 2h Swing	1			

#138 ☆ The Abduction of Fran

M	R	Exercise	Sets	Reps	Rest	Note
SEQUENCE	2	^{B13} Pull-Up	1	12	Brief, +5min after round	Each round AQAP
		^{C11} KB Thruster, 2KB	1	12		
		^{B13} Pull-Up	1	9		
		^{C11} KB Thruster, 2KB	1	9		
		^{B13} Pull-Up	1	6		
		^{C11} KB Thruster, 2KB	1	6		

WEEK 47

#139 ☆ The Ministry of Funny Walks

M	R	Exercise	Sets	Reps	Rest	Note
SEQUENCE	4	G01 Model Walk	1	15-20m each	15-20s/set, +1 min/round	
		G03 Rooster Walk	1			
		C18 Lunge Walk	1			
		G02 Chaplin Walk	1			
		G05 Bear Walk	1			
		D09 Hzt Frog Jump	1			
		G04 Crab Walk	1			
		D11 Sprunglauf	1			
		G06 Wheelbarrow	1			

#140 ☆ Fit for the Cross 2

M	R	Exercise	Sets	Reps	Rest	Note
		C20 KB Lunge Walk, 2KB	As req.	70	As req.	In sequence, AQAP. Break up into manageable sets.
		E15 Sit-Up	As req.	60	As req.	
		F13 KB 2h Swing	As req.	50	As req.	
		E21 Hanging Leg Raise	As req.	40	As req.	
		B13 Pull-Up	As req.	30	As req.	
		A08 Diamond Push-Up	As req.	20	As req.	

#141 ☆ Best Buddies

M	R	Exercise	Sets	Reps	Rest	Note
SEQ.	3	G06 Wheelbarrow	2	20m each	1min each	
		G11 Buddy Carry	2			
		G12 Buddy Pull	2			
		G13 Reverse Buddy Pull	2			

WEEK 48

#142 ☆ Short Cycle AMRAP

M	R	Exercise	Sets	Reps	Rest	Note
CIRC.	AMRAP	B12 Chin-Up	1	5	Brief	AMRAP 30min
		F16 KB High Swing	1	5		
		A18 **Hanging Dips**	1	5		
		D06 Vertical Jump	1	5		

#143 ☆ Temple of the Body

M	R	Exercise	Sets	Reps	Rest	Note
		B13 Pull-Up	As req.	25	Brief	
		D08 Box Jump	As req.	25		
		A06 Push-Up	As req.	50		
		C05 Hindu Squat	As req.	50		
		F08 SL Glute Bridge	As req.	25 ea.		
		E22 Inverted Ab Tuck	As req.	50		
		C15 Step-Up Jump	As req.	50		
		B08 Inverted Row	As req.	50		
		C18 Lunge Walk	As req.	50		
		C03 Air Squat	As req.	50		
		A08 Diamond Push-Up	As req.	25		
		B12 Chin-Up	As req.	25		

#144 ☆ Rehab

M	R	Exercise	Sets	Reps	Rest	Note
SEQUENCE	6	F01 Hurdles	1 ea.	6 ea.	Brief/ set, +2min/ round	Slow to moderate pace; Don't rush. Move about between rounds.
		C01 Calf Raise	1	6		
		C06 Prisoner Squat	1	6		
		F03 Down Dog / Up Dog	1	6		
		B02 Superman Row	1	6		
		A06 Push-Up	1	6		
		E06 Bird Dog Plank	1	6		
		C18 Lunge Walk	1	6		

WEEK 49

#145 ☆

M	R	Exercise	Sets	Reps	Rest	Note
SS	15	G07 KB Farmer Walk	1	20m	Brief	Don't rush.
		A08 Diamond Push-Up	1	5		
SS	5	G10 KB Pick-Up Walk	1	10		
		E20 Flat Leg Raise	1	10		

#146 ☆ The Alternate 300

M	R	Exercise	Sets	Reps	Rest	Note
		F17 KB Clean, 2KB	As req.	25	Brief, as req.	Go for a long first set of each. Brief rest, but don't rush.
		A18 Hanging Dips	As req.	50		
		C15 Step-Up Jump	As req.	50		
		E22 Inverted Ab Tuck	As req.	50		
		C07 KB Goblet Squat	As req.	50		
		E18 KB Russian Twist	As req.	50		
		B12 Chin-Up	As req.	25		

#147 ☆ Prof. Tabata's Curse

M	R	Exercise	Sets	Reps	Rest	Note
		A17 Seated Dips	8	20s	10s/ set, +2min/ exercise	
		G14 Run-In-Place	8	20s		
		E07 Mtn. Climber	8	20s		
		B07 KB High Pull	8	20s		Alt./ set
		D05 Vertical Frog Jump	8	20s		

WEEK 50

#148 ☆ Long Cycle

M	R	Exercise	Sets	Reps	Rest	Note
SEQUENCE	10	^{F16} KB High Swing	1	10 each	n/a	
		^{F17} KB Clean, R	1			
		^{F17} KB Clean, L	1			
		^{D13} Push-Up Burpee	1			
		^{E08} Everest Mtn. Climber	1	20	2min	

#149 ☆ Circuit No. 3

M	R	Exercise	Sets	Reps	Rest	Note
CIRCUIT	2	^{F01} Hurdles	1 ea.	30s/ set	20s/ set, +2min/ round	Fast
		^{D05} Vertical Frog Jump	2			
		^{B02} Superman Row	2			
		^{D04} Kick-Back Jump	2			
		^{E03} Low Plank	2			30s or ALAP
		^{E06} Bird Dog Plank	2			Slow
		^{D02} Shuffle Jump	2			
		^{B04} Standing Band Row	2			
		^{C15} Step-Up Jump	2			

#150 ☆ TEST, The BW500

M	R	Exercise	Sets	Reps	Rest	Note
		^{B08} Inverted Row	As req.	25	As req.	AQAP For total time
		^{D12} Burpee	As req.	50		
		^{A06} Push-Up	As req.	50		
		^{C03} Air Squat	As req.	100		
		^{E08} Everest Mtn. Climber	As req.	100		
		^{F06} Glute Bridge	As req.	100		
		^{E14} Rower Sit-Up	As req.	50		
		^{B08} Inverted Row	As req.	25		

4. EXERCISES

A. Push Exercises

A01   Band Push

Introduced WO#	10
Occurrences in program:	10
Primary muscle groups:	Chest; Arms

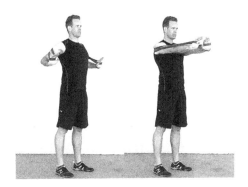

Wrap the resistance band behind your upper back and put your hands through the ends of the loop. You could also anchor the band around a light pole or similar. Start the push at the lower part of the chest muscles, squeezing your shoulder blades gently together. Push forward until your hands meet. Slowly return to start and repeat. Keep your shoulders low and the midsection tight throughout.

A02   Scapular Push-Up

Introduced WO#	11
Occurrences in program:	4
Primary muscle groups:	Upper back; Shoulders

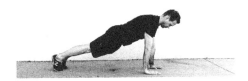
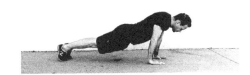

This is quite subtle: Start out in the upper position of the push-up. Your hands and toes should be touching the floor, and your body should form a straight line from your shoulders to your ankles. The main goal here is to squeeze your shoulder blades together. Your chest will move towards the floor, but your back should stay straight, and your elbows should not bend. Push back up a little bit past the starting position. Keep the neck straight and relaxed.

A03   Half Push-Up

Introduced WO#	7
Occurrences in program:	5
Primary muscle groups:	Chest; Arms

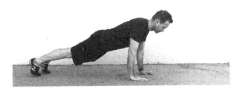
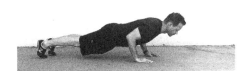

The Half Push-Up is an intermediate variety of the regular Push-Up (A06); it is a little less strenuous. Most people can manage this even if the regular push-up is too challenging. Start from the standard push-up position, and lower yourself approximately half way to the ground. Push back up and repeat. Keep your body straight and the midsection tight. Avoid flaring the elbows out.

A04   Negative Push-Up

Introduced WO#   22
Occurrences in program: 2
Primary muscle groups: Chest; Arms

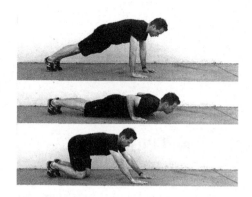

The Negative Push-Up is an intermediate step on the way to achieving a full push-up. The focus is on the negative part of the move, i.e. on the way down. Keep the midsection tight and straight. Try to descend slowly and stay in control throughout. To get back up, put your knees to the ground. Hinge at the hips and slide back and up.

A05   Incline Push-Up

Introduced WO#   56
Occurrences in program: 1
Primary muscle groups: Chest; Arms

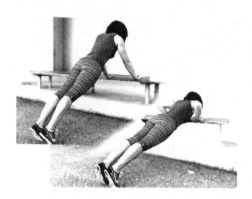

Push-Ups with your hands on an elevated surface, such as a bench, chair, stairs or low wall; less demanding than a regular push-up. A good place to start if you have not done much (upper body) exercise in the past. This exercise can be fully modified to suit your level; the easiest form would be to simply lean in with your palms flat against a wall and push slowly away. As you get stronger, move gradually down toward the ground; a flight of stairs is convenient.

A06   Push-Up

Introduced WO#   1
Occurrences in program: 46
Primary muscle groups: Chest; Arms

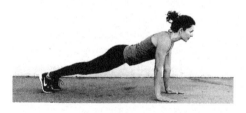

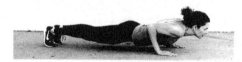

From a high plank position, lower yourself until the chest very nearly touches the floor. Push back up and repeat, keeping the body completely straight and rigid throughout - no slouching or sticking the butt up. The hand position should be approximately shoulder width and the elbows should not flare out to the sides much as you lower yourself – that will hurt your shoulders. Approx. 45° angle between the upper arm and spine is generally good. Substitute with A03-A05 until you can perform correctly.

A07   Decline Push-Up

Introduced WO#   82
Occurrences in program: 2
Primary muscle groups: Chest; Arms

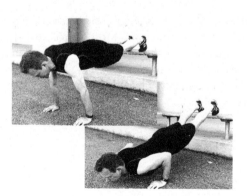

Push-Ups with your feet on an elevated surface, such as a bench, chair, stairs or low wall. This is more demanding than a regular push-up and shifts more of the load onto the upper chest muscles and front of the shoulders. You can use this as an alternate exercise to A06 for variation.

A08   Diamond Push-Up

Introduced WO#   77
Occurrences in program: 7
Primary muscle groups: Chest; Arms

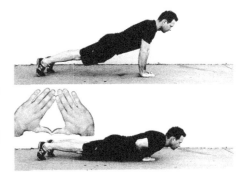

The name refers to the hand stance: Place your hands so that your index fingers and thumbs touch and they'll form a diamond shape. This will shift a greater portion of the load onto your triceps and make it more demanding. This exercise is a necessary step toward being able to do one-arm push-ups; however, while you're working on accomplishing this exercise it is beneficial to also complement with other variations of the push-up.

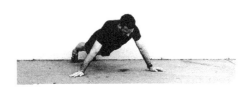

A09   Wide Push-Up

Introduced WO#   89
Occurrences in program: 3
Primary muscle groups: Chest; Arms
                                  (chest dominant)

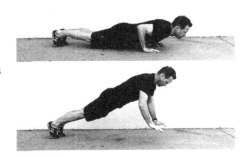

Push-ups with a wide hand-stance. This shifts more of the load unto your chest and shoulders. The palms will need to be turned out a little to avoid putting too much strain on the elbows.

A10   Plyo Push-Up

Introduced WO#   91
Occurrences in program: 3
Primary muscle groups: Chest; Arms

Plyo is short for *plyometric*, in other words a forceful, explosive move. In practical terms, this means that as you do the push-up, you thrust your arms forward hard and fast enough to lift your hands of the ground. Clapping may be introduced for the sheer spectacle of it. Landing on your face is not quite as cool.

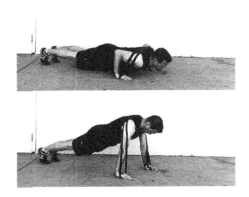

A11   Band Push-Up

Introduced WO#   84
Occurrences in program: 3
Primary muscle groups: Chest; Arms

Wrap the resistance band across your upper back. Grab the ends. Do a push-up. This allows you to add some extra resistance to the push-up.

A12   Walking Push-Up

Introduced WO#   70
Occurrences in program: 5
Primary muscle groups: Chest; Arms

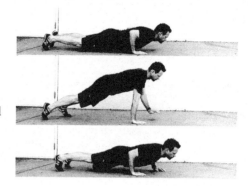

Start from the push-up high position, but with one hand slightly in front of the other. Do a push-up. As you come back up, move the rear hand to the front and do another push up. Your legs will need to follow. This should add up to a slow, forward walk. Kind of like a lunge walk. But on your hands. Right? Anyhow.

A13   KB Floor Press

Introduced WO#   56
Occurrences in program: 3
Primary muscle groups: Chest; Arms

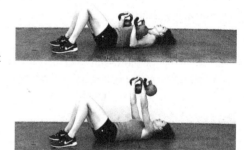

Lie down flat on your back. Bend your knees to 90 degrees with your feet flat on the ground. Grab a kettlebell in each hand with your forearms firmly against the lower ribcage and your elbows on the ground – rolling to the side may help you get the bells to the chest. When both bells are secure and stable, determinedly press them straight up, bringing your hands close together. Return to the chest in a controlled motion.

A14   KB Press

Introduced WO#   20
Occurrences in program: 8
Primary muscle groups: Shoulders; Arms

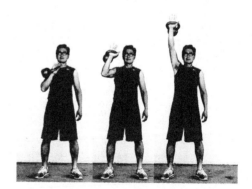

From the rack position (KB resting against the upper arm and thumb against the collar bone), press the bell overhead to a straight arm. Avoid dipping or pushing with your legs. Keep your midsection tight – that's the foundation you're pressing from.

A15   KB OH Static

Introduced WO#   65
Occurrences in program: 2
Primary muscle groups: Shoulders

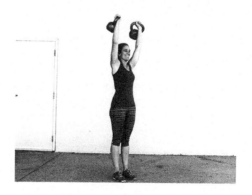

Well… From the rack position, press the bell or bells all the way overhead to straight arm(s). Keep tension in your midsection. Hold. Hold. Hold. Etc.

A16   KB Halo

Introduced WO#   47
Occurrences in program: 2
Primary muscle groups: Shoulders; Chest; Arms

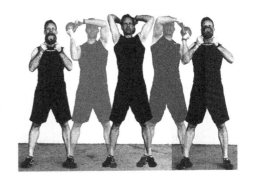

Yeah, OK – strictly speaking it's not a push. Nor a pull. But it does work all the little support muscles that are very important for both, and opens up restrictions in the shoulders. Hold the KB with both hands and the bell up in front of your face. Slowly circle your head with the KB, keeping it at roughly the same level throughout. Make sure that you work both directions equally. This is excellent as a warm-up exercise.

A17   Seated Dips

Introduced WO#   2
Occurrences in program: 16
Primary muscle groups: Chest; Triceps; Shoulders

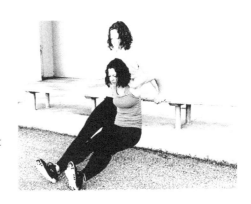

Dips mainly work the backside of the upper arm (triceps), front shoulder and chest. With your heels on the ground and your legs extended, rest your bodyweight on your hands at hip height. Dip slowly down to about 90 degrees bend in the elbow, then extend the arms. You can go lower, but it'll put a lot of strain on the front of the shoulder, so be careful.

A18   Hanging Dips

Introduced WO#   142
Occurrences in program: 3
Primary muscle groups: Chest; Triceps; Shoulders

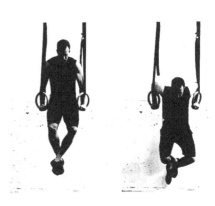

Dips mainly work the backside of the upper arm (triceps), front shoulder and chest. Hanging freely from a double bar or rings, rest your bodyweight on your hands at hip height. Dip slowly down to about 90 degrees bend in the elbow and then extend the arms. You can go lower, but it will put a lot of strain on the front of the shoulder, so be careful.

B. Pull Exercises

B01   Bat Wings

Introduced WO#	2
Occurrences in program:	6
Primary muscle groups:	Upper back

The objective is to activate the scapular muscles. Stand up straight with your shoulders back and low. Hold your arms up with the upper arm straight out from the shoulder and the lower arm up, i.e. 90 degrees bend at the elbow. Slowly squeeze the shoulder blades together hard. Relax and repeat.

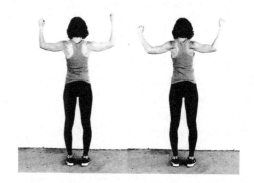

B02   Superman Row

Introduced WO#	2
Occurrences in program:	16
Primary muscle groups:	Upper back; Lower back

Lie face down on the ground with the arms stretched out in front of you. Tighten your glutes and back and lift the legs and chest off the ground – this is the Superman-part. Now pull the arms back and squeeze your shoulder blades together hard; that's the row. Reverse and repeat.

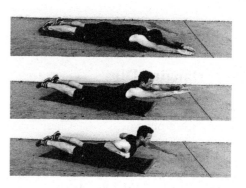

B03   Seated Band Row

Introduced WO#	7
Occurrences in program:	10
Primary muscle groups:	Upper back; Arms

Sit down with your legs straight out in front of you. Position the band under your feet. Grab the ends. Pull to the lower rib cage. Keep your back straight and squeeze the shoulder blades together when pulling. You should feel the muscles between the shoulder blades almost cramping. Slowly relax and repeat.

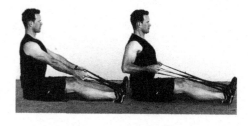

B04   Standing Band Row

Introduced WO#	33
Occurrences in program:	8
Primary muscle groups:	Upper back; Arms

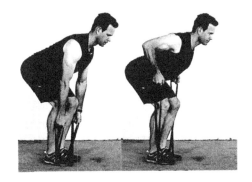

Stand over the center of the band with feet shoulder-width apart. Bend slightly at the knees and hinge at the hips, keeping your hips back. Tighten your midsection and keep the lower back flat. Grasp the ends of band and pull toward the lower ribcage. Try to squeeze your shoulder blades together in the top position.

B05   KB Supported Row

Introduced WO#	17
Occurrences in program:	10
Primary muscle groups:	Upper back; Arms

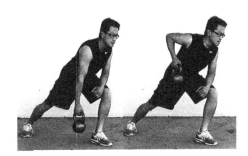

Stand with one leg forward and bent, and the rear leg straight. Place a kettlebell next to the inner ankle of the front leg. Lean forward and support your forearm just above the knee of the front leg, grab the handle of the kettlebell, and pull to the lower ribcage.

B06   KB Renegade Row

Introduced WO#	50
Occurrences in program:	8
Primary muscle groups:	Upper back; Arms; Core

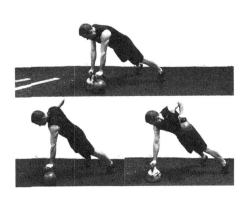

The Renegade Row can be very taxing and is an outstanding core stability exercise. Assume the push-up position with your hands on the handles of two kettlebells. If your KBs are unstable, you may need to lay one of them flat, put your hand on the body of the bell, and work one side at a time. For stability, use a slightly wider foot position than normal. Tighten your midsection hard. Alternately pull one bell to the lower ribcage. Try to avoid twisting at the hips.

B07   KB High Pull

Introduced WO#	38
Occurrences in program:	8
Primary muscle groups:	Upper back; Posterior chain; Arms

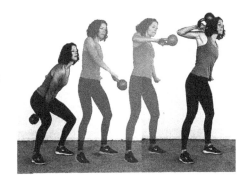

This lift starts like a KB Clean (F17). As you swing the bell up, however, you allow it to travel a little higher and slightly more to the side. Pull the arm back as far as it goes, letting the bell travel just over and outside of your shoulder. Immediately push forward against the handle and swing the bell down between your legs. Watching a few YouTube videos is recommended.

B08   Inverted Row

Introduced WO#   1
Occurrences in program: 26
Primary muscle groups: Upper back; Arms

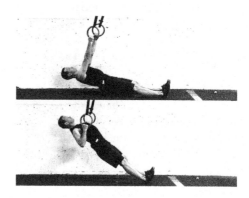

Pull to the lower rib cage and squeeze the shoulder blades together. Inverted Rows can be adapted to your individual level by adjusting the angle; the more horizontal your body is, the heavier it gets. You could also bend at the knees to make it easier. The benchmark is being fully horizontal in the lower (extended arm) position. Elevating your feet will make it more challenging.

B09   Dead Hang Low

Introduced WO#   43
Occurrences in program: 3
Primary muscle groups: Shoulders; Arms

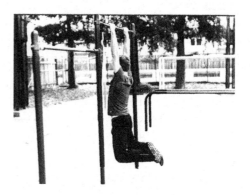

This exercise is one end point of the pull-up, and will help develop the strength needed to perform a pull-up or additional reps. The low variety strengthens the grip and shoulder girdle. As you might expect, it is static; in other words, you just hang in there (pun intended!) without moving.

B10   Dead Hang High

Introduced WO#   50
Occurrences in program: 6
Primary muscle groups: Upper back; Arms

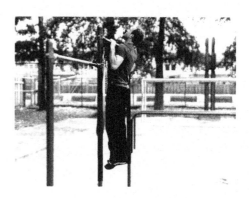

The high Dead Hang is the other end point of the pull-up, and will help develop the strength needed to perform a pull-up or additional reps. The high variety strengthens the grip, upper arms and upper back. As you might expect, it is also static. Somewhat obviously, you could also introduce a dead hang variety anywhere between the High and Low endpoints if you wish to address a particular weakness.

B11   Negative Pull-Up

Introduced WO#   61
Occurrences in program: 4
Primary muscle groups: Upper back; Arms

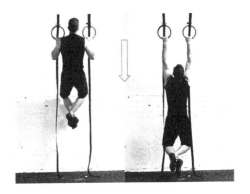

A Negative Pull-Up (or Chin-Up) is a one-way street: You only move from the upper position to the lower position. By inference, you may need a stool or something like that to get up there… Hold back and try to control the motion on your way down. We tend to be a little stronger when extending the arm, so this exercise is helpful when training to achieve a regular pull-up.

B12   Chin-Up

Introduced WO#   63
Occurrences in program: 8
Primary muscle groups: Upper back; Arms

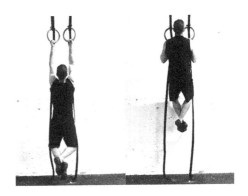

Terminology varies: We consider the Chin-Up to be a Pull-Up with an underhand grip, i.e. palms facing you. The grip is often slightly narrower than for the regular Pull-Up, to avoid straining the elbow too much. The Chin-Up puts more of the load away from the back muscles and onto the biceps, and is somewhat less demanding overall.

B13   Pull-Up

Introduced WO#   47
Occurrences in program: 24
Primary muscle groups: Upper back; Arms

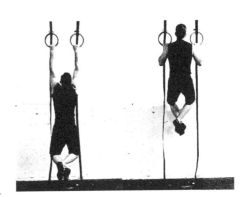

We all know this one, right? As far as we're concerned, Pull-Ups are done with an overhand grip, i.e. the back of the hand faces you. Grip the bar slightly wider than shoulder width; a couple of inches narrower can help you get a bit higher, though. A wider grip will work the back muscles more, but may also strain the shoulders. Try to get high, almost to where the chest touches the bar, and then lower yourself to very nearly fully extended arms; the shoulders and elbows should always be kept in tension, as should your midsection. Substitute with B11-B12 or use a resistance band to assist in the lift until you can do 3 consecutive reps.

C. Squat and Lunge Exercises

C01   Calf Raise

Introduced WO#   39
Occurrences in program: 5
Primary muscle groups: Legs (calves)

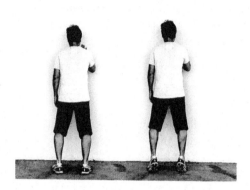

Stand with the balls of your feet on the edge of a step or flat on the ground. Stand tall, i.e. chest held high and mid-section in tension. Lift yourself up on your toes, hold for a second, then lower yourself back down. This exercise mainly works the thick calf muscles. For a more challenging variety, do it one leg at a time, or add external load, e.g. kettlebells.

C02   Air Bench

Introduced WO#   2
Occurrences in program: 7
Primary muscle groups: Legs (thighs)

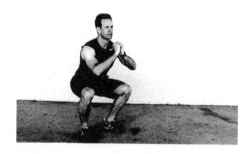

Air Bench is essentially a static Air Squat (C03), i.e. keep the thighbone roughly parallel to the ground. Foot position may be a little wider than standard squat position, i.e. just over shoulder width. Sit there and suffer, it is good for you.

C03   Air Squat

Introduced WO#   1
Occurrences in program: 17
Primary muscle groups: Legs

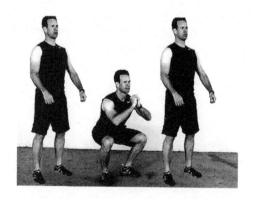

Squatting is fundamental. Every healthy toddler in the world knows how to do it correctly; unfortunately, most of us grow up and forget. The squat is done with the feet about shoulder-width a part and toes pointed slightly (and evenly) out; knees follow the same direction. The Air Squat turn-around point is a little higher than in a full squat: Thighbone approximately parallel to the ground. Keep the back straight and midsection tight.

C04   Squat Jump

Introduced WO#	45
Occurrences in program:	12
Primary muscle groups:	Legs

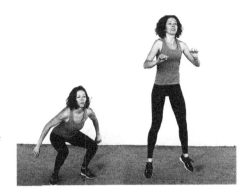

The Squat Jump is pretty much the same as a more forcefully executed, explosive Air Squat. Make sure that you land on slightly bent legs to absorb the shock. Focus on squatting properly down: The optimal depth for jumping is actually not quite as deep as the Air Squat depth (thighbone parallel to ground), so it's easy to slip away from the Squat part of this when doing a longer series. Stay focused. You're not supposed to jump very high, just a small lift-off.

C05   Hindu Squat

Introduced WO#	8
Occurrences in program:	9
Primary muscle groups:	Legs

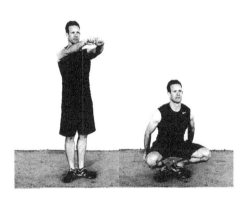

Hindu Squats differ from regular squats by requiring you to go up on your toes in the lower position. This can be a little demanding in terms of balance, but it's also easier than regular squats if you have hip or ankle flexibility issues. Stand up straight with your heels close together and toes pointed out. Bend your legs to lower yourself into a squat while allowing the heels to lift. Make sure the knees point in the same direction as your toes, i.e. outward.

C06   Prisoner Squat

Introduced WO#	39
Occurrences in program:	9
Primary muscle groups:	Legs

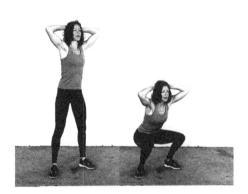

The Prisoner Squat is not that different from an Air Squat, but the hands are placed behind your head with the elbows flared out – i.e. like a POW… It actually helps you maintain posture better.

C07   KB Goblet Squat

Introduced WO#	23
Occurrences in program:	11
Primary muscle groups:	Legs; Core

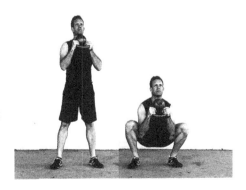

Hold a kettlebell by the handle with both hands in front of the chest. Squat down deep, keeping your back straight. If you notice your lower back rounding, don't go any deeper. Stand back up. Foot position should be just wide enough to allow your elbows to fit between your knees. This also requires that the toes are pointed outward slightly, i.e. the knees should travel in the same direction as the feet are pointing.

C08   KB H2H Sumo Squat

Introduced WO#   59
Occurrences in program: 3
Primary muscle groups: Legs; Core

Whether to call this a squat or a deadlift is a little arbitrary. You assume a sumo stance, i.e. wider than the normal squat position. Toes are pointed well out. Holding the kettlebell with one hand, squat down until the bell touches the ground, then stand back up straight. H2H means hand-to-hand, i.e. switch hands every time you straighten up or touch down – whichever works for you. Make it fast and fluid.

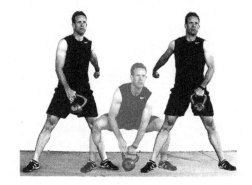

C09   KB Front Squat

Introduced WO#   35
Occurrences in program: 4
Primary muscle groups: Legs; Core

Clean one or two kettlebells to the rack position (F17). Keep your core tight and squat until your hips are below the knees. Foot position should be wide enough that two bells can fit between them on the ground, with toes pointed slightly out.

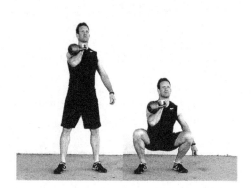

C10   KB OH Squat

Introduced WO#   76
Occurrences in program: 5
Primary muscle groups: Legs; Core: Shoulders

You start with the bell overhead, i.e. you need to clean and press the bell first (F18). Feet just over shoulder-width apart. Squat down, maintaining the bell locked out overhead on a straight arm. As you squat, you'll need to twist your upper body a little to be able to keep the arm vertical. Return to the starting position.

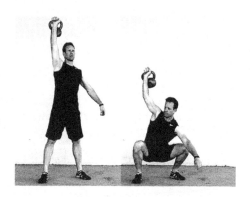

C11   KB Thruster

Introduced WO#   98
Occurrences in program: 6
Primary muscle groups: Legs; Core: Shoulders; Arms

As much a press as a squat, "Thrusters" is a CrossFit staple that simply means the combination of a fast front squat and push-press. In other words: Rack the kettlebell(s), squat down, then explosively straighten up. As you near the top position, push up hard and extend the kettlebells on straight arms.

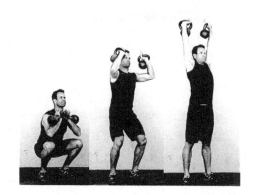

C12   Sk8 Squat

Introduced WO#   22
Occurrences in program: 11
Primary muscle groups: Legs; Hips

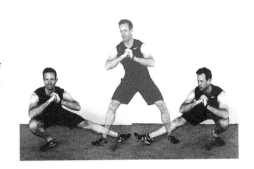

Move from side to side in a skating motion with the feet wide apart. In the lower position, one leg should be straight and resting on the heel, whereas the other is well bent and resting on a flat foot. Apart from flipping between flat foot and heel, the foot position should not change.

C13   Bulgarian Split Squat

Introduced WO#   74
Occurrences in program: 5
Primary muscle groups: Legs; Glutes

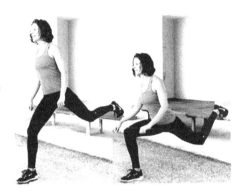

Sometimes referred to as RFESS = Rear Foot Elevated Split Squat. Basically a lunge-in-place with the rear foot on an elevated surface. The rear foot should only rest there, not bear any weight. In a controlled manner, bend the front knee to 90° and then come back up. The shin should be close to vertical in the lower position, with the knee not moving too far in front of the ankle joint. Hold a couple of kettlebells if you'd like prolonged soreness.

C14   Step-Up

Introduced WO#   2
Occurrences in program: 10
Primary muscle groups: Legs; Glutes

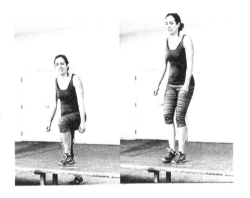

Stand facing a bench, step or platform. Place foot of first leg on bench. Stand on bench by extending hip and knee of first leg and place foot of second leg on bench. Step down with second leg by flexing hip and knee of first leg. Return to original standing position by placing foot of first leg to floor. Repeat sequence with opposite leg. Keep the torso upright during the exercise. The leading knee should point in the same direction as the foot throughout.

C15   Step-Up Jump

Introduced WO#   33
Occurrences in program: 10
Primary muscle groups: Legs; Glutes

Nearly identical to the standard Step-Up described above, but you drive the front leg down more forcefully so that you lift off from the ground. In mid-air, switch the legs so the down-step and following forceful up-step is done with the other leg.

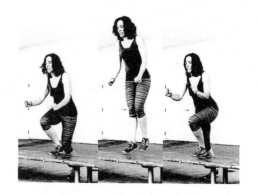

C16   Static Lunge

Introduced WO#   20
Occurrences in program: 4
Primary muscle groups: Legs; Glutes

Static Lunges work your glutes and quads, and they help develop stamina in these muscle groups. Drop into a lunge with your rear leg knee just off the ground. The front leg shin bone should be close to vertical. Stay. Fell the burn.

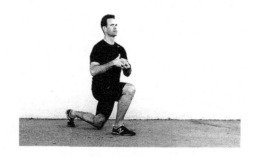

C17   Bwd Lunge

Introduced WO#   17
Occurrences in program: 9
Primary muscle groups: Legs; Glutes

The Lunge is essentially a long, really deep stride. In the lower position, the front knee should be bent to about 90 degrees, with the calf bone roughly vertical. The knee of the rear leg should be behind the body's centerline, and very close to the ground. We prefer stepping *back* in a Backward Lunge; this makes it easier to control the stability of the forward knee. Return to standing. If you simply stay in the lunge position for some time, that's a Static Lunge (C16, above).

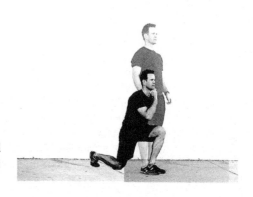

C18   Lunge Walk

Introduced WO#   39
Occurrences in program: 13
Primary muscle groups: Legs; Glutes

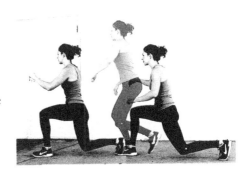

Rather self-explanatory, don't you think? Move fluently from one lunge to the next by taking an elongated, deep stride forward. Continue for the required time or number of repetitions. Add kettlebells for extra resistance if you feel like it (ref. C20).

C19   KB OH Bwd Lunge

Introduced WO#   32
Occurrences in program: 4
Primary muscle groups: Legs; Glutes; Core; Shoulders

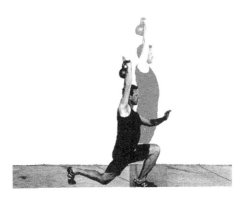

"Kettlebell Overhead, Backward Lunge". Start by standing straight and press the kettlebell over your head, locking out the elbow. The bell should be kept on a straight arm throughout. Take a long, deep step back, bringing your rear knee almost to the ground (Backward Lunge, C17). Return to standing. The front leg is normally on the side holding the bell.

C20   KB Lunge Walk

Introduced WO#   92
Occurrences in program: 4
Primary muscle groups: Legs; Glutes; Core; Shoulders

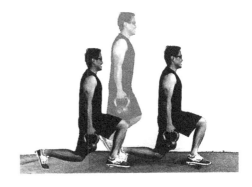

A Lunge Walk (C18), while carrying a kettlebell in each hand. Yes, that makes it quite a bit harder than the regular Lunge Walk.

D. Jump Exercises

D01   Jumping Jack

Introduced WO#   17
Occurrences in program: 5
Primary muscle groups: Legs; Hips; Shoulders

Jumping Jacks is an old favorite that pops up in many workout regimes. A light and quick jump with large motion patterns, it's a great cardio-dominant exercise with limited impact forces.

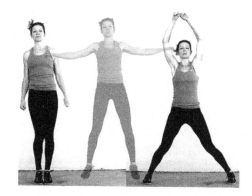

D02   Shuffle Jump

Introduced WO#   7
Occurrences in program: 8
Primary muscle groups: Legs

The Shuffle Jump is a light and quick jump performed with no forward motion. On the balls of your feet from a split leg stance, do a light jump to change leg position. Repeat instantly. Swing your arms in big motions to provide counterbalance. Similar to the Lunge Jump but nowhere near as deep or powerful, it most resembles the motion in classical Nordic (cross-country) skiing. The Shuffle Jump can be done for high reps and you should be able to do at least 2 per second.

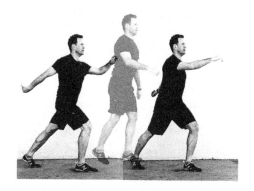

D03   Zig-Zag Jump

Introduced WO#   26
Occurrences in program: 6
Primary muscle groups: Legs

The Zig Zag Jump is a light, quick, sideways jump with no forward motion. Stay on the balls of your feet and do a light sideways jump with both legs together. To maintain focus, it is nice to have something on the ground to jump across, e.g. a kettlebell or a bag.

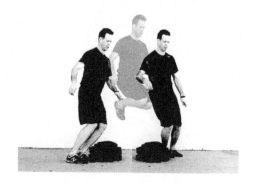

D04   Kick-Back Jump

Introduced WO#   10
Occurrences in program: 7
Primary muscle groups: Legs; Core

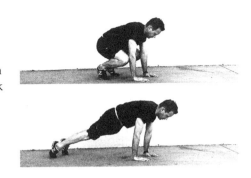

The Kick-Back Jump is one half of the beloved Burpee. Crouch down with
your palms flat on the ground; jump back into the Push-Up or High Plank
position; jump forward back into a crouch. Repeat. This can be done in
quick succession for a high number of reps to achieve a solid cardio/
respiratory punch.

D05   Vertical Frog Jump

Introduced WO#   33
Occurrences in program: 6
Primary muscle groups: Legs

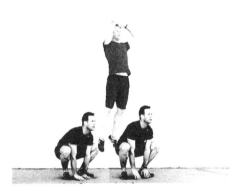

The Vertical Frog Jump is a deep, moderate to high-power, vertical jump
with no forward motion. It's not all that different from a Vertical Jump,
but you go deeper, touching the ground with your palms, and you push off
with less than maximum capacity. Try to land softly, dampening the
touchdown with a deep flex of the legs as you crouch down.

D06   Vertical Jump

Introduced WO#   61
Occurrences in program: 4
Primary muscle groups: Legs

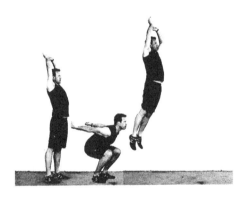

The Vertical Jump is a maximum (or near maximum) effort jump with no
forward motion. Drive your arms back down fast as you bend your knees
moderately into a high squat. Use the momentum to thrust your arms up
high as you extend your legs forcefully. Jump as high as you can and try to
land softly on the balls of your feet, flexing the legs slightly to dampen the
impact. Don't squat too deep, it'll reduce your ability to generate power.

D07   Tuck jump

Introduced WO#   56
Occurrences in program: 5
Primary muscle groups: Legs; Core

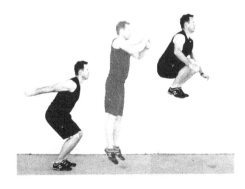

The Tuck Jump is a powerful and fast jump. Jump straight up, driving the
arms up. As you do, pull your knees up toward your chest, i.e. tuck. Land
softly on the balls of your feet. Try to spend as little time on the ground as
possible; bounce straight back up. The Tuck Jump packs a serious punch
and will leave you out of breath in no time.

D08   Box Jump

Introduced WO#   67
Occurrences in program: 13
Primary muscle groups: Legs

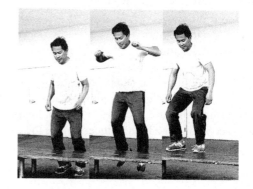

Jump. Onto a box, or something similar. It is advisable that whatever you land on is sturdy and stable; a cardboard box will not do… Jump back down and try to land softly. Step back down only if you have bad knees. Drive your arms up for the lift-off, and back when you jump down. Work on finding a good rhythm to the jump; you should be able to do multiple reps with minimal time spent on the ground.

D09   Horizontal Frog Jump

Introduced WO#   46
Occurrences in program: 6
Primary muscle groups: Legs

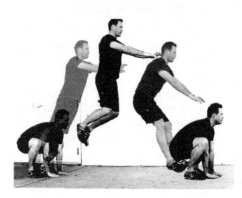

The Horizontal Frog Jump is a powerful, long jump that requires some experience with jumping – it's very similar to a standing broad jump. This can be hard on your knees if you're not prepared. From the frog position (squatting with your palms flat on the ground), extend your legs hard and fast while you drive your arms up. Extend fully and try to land softly on the balls of your feet, back into the frog position. Landing on your heels on a hard surface will ruin them.

D10   Lunge Jump

Introduced WO#   76
Occurrences in program: 5
Primary muscle groups: Legs

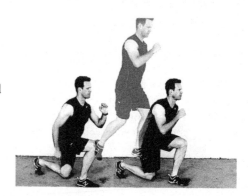

Descend into the lunge position with the rear knee close to the ground and your forward knee bent at a 90-degree angle. Jump up off the ground slightly, and quickly switch the position of your feet in mid-air. Lend back into the lunge position with the other knee forward. Keep your torso straight throughout the exercise.

D11   Sprunglauf

Introduced WO#   46
Occurrences in program: 6
Primary muscle groups: Legs

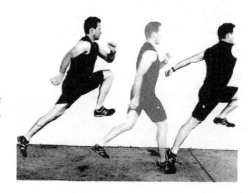

The term is German and literally translates to "leap run". In other words: You execute a series of fast, long, bouncing leaps. The focus is more on the length of each stride than the height, although you do need some lift-off to make it work. It should be fluent and fast; spend as little time on the ground as possible. This is hard on the leg muscles and ligaments, so be careful and well warmed up.

D12   Burpee

Introduced WO#	1
Occurrences in program:	20
Primary muscle groups:	Legs; Core

A particularly nasty torture method applied by crossfitters, PTs, and the army alike, occasionally referred to as cardio purgatory. Crouch down; kick feet back into the plank position; jump back to the crouch position; then jump straight up. Repeat ad nauseam. The Burpee is a combination of a Kick-Back Jump (D04) and Vertical Frog Jump (D05).

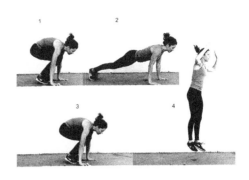

D13   Push-Up Burpee

Introduced WO#	63
Occurrences in program:	5
Primary muscle groups:	Legs; Chest; Core

Burpees as described above (D12), but including a Push-Up (A06) in the kick-back position. This seems to be the standard CrossFit Burpee.

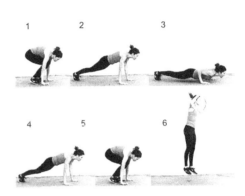

D14   Bastard Burpee

Introduced WO#	63
Occurrences in program:	2
Primary muscle groups:	Legs; Chest; Core

Push-Up Burpees (D13) where you jump straight up in a Tuck Jump (D07). No sweat.

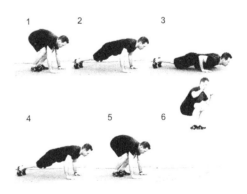

E. Anterior Chain Exercises

E01   High Plank

Introduced WO#   47
Occurrences in program: 3
Primary muscle groups: Anterior chain

Assume the initial position of a standard push-up. Stay there. Be conscious of keeping a tight midsection, and do not allow your hips to sag. The High Plank is slightly less demanding than the standard Plank. After a while you should feel a burn develop in your straight abdominal muscles. To increase difficulty, walk your hands forward.

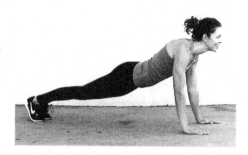

E02   Plank

Introduced WO#   2
Occurrences in program: 10
Primary muscle groups: Anterior chain

Get into a prone position on the floor, supporting your weight on your toes and your forearms. Your arms are bent and directly below the shoulder. Keep your body straight at all times, and hold this position as long as possible. Focus on keeping tension in the abdominal muscles. To increase difficulty, an arm or leg can be raised.

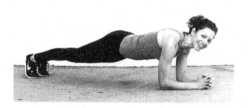

E03   Low Plank

Introduced WO#   33
Occurrences in program: 6
Primary muscle groups: Anterior chain; Chest

Essentially the lower end of the push-up; the turn-around point. Chest 2 inches off the ground. Keep the load on your chest and arms with a ramrod-straight midsection. Stay there and suffer.

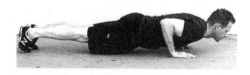

E04 Side Plank

Introduced WO#	2
Occurrences in program:	9
Primary muscle groups:	Lateral chain

Works your oblique abdominal muscles and helps stabilize your spine. Lie on your side and support your body between your forearm and your feet. The spine and hips should be straight. Hold position. Raising an arm to the heavens and praying to your chosen deity for relief is optional.

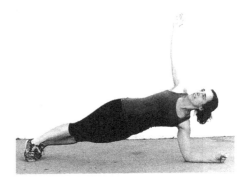

E05 X-Kick High Plank

Introduced WO#	64
Occurrences in program:	6
Primary muscle groups:	Anterior chain

From the High Plank position, move one knee to the opposite elbow in a controlled, deliberate manner. The forward foot does not touch the ground. Return to start. Repeat on the other side. Try to avoid twisting the hips.

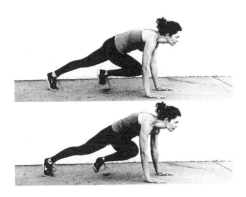

E06 Bird Dog Plank

Introduced WO#	33
Occurrences in program:	8
Primary muscle groups:	Anterior chain; Posterior chain

Starting from the High Plank position, slowly lift one arm and the opposite leg off the ground. Keep arms and legs straight throughout. Move slowly and maintain your balance. Do not let your hips sag.

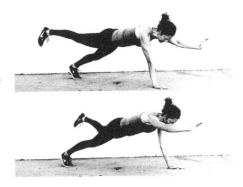

E07 Mtn. Climber

Introduced WO#	45
Occurrences in program:	7
Primary muscle groups:	Anterior chain; Shoulders; Legs

The Mountain Climber is a staple. Start from the High Plank or initial Push-Up position. Bring one leg forward to a split leg stance. Do a small jump to switch foot position, and then immediately repeat without rest. Stay on the balls of your feet. The motion should be light and quick with just the briefest touchdown.

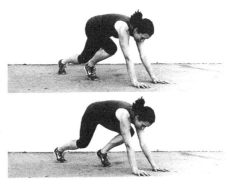

E08   Everest Mtn. Climber

Introduced WO#   1
Occurrences in program: 18
Primary muscle groups: Anterior chain; Shoulders; Legs

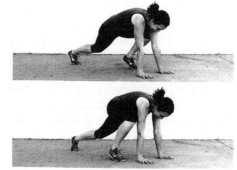

Very similar to the standard Mountain Climber, except that you'll pull
your legs further forward so the knee ends up outside the elbow. This
forces the hips to open up and the pelvis to rotate. This makes the Everest
is more strenuous than the regular Mountain Climber, but it also increases
hip mobility – much needed for most of us. The rotation can be hard on
your lower back; if you experience lower back pain you may want to stick
to regular Mtn. Climbers (E07).

E09   Crunch

Introduced WO#   2
Occurrences in program: 9
Primary muscle groups: Abdominals

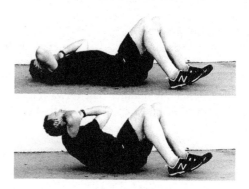

Lie down flat on your back, legs at 90 degrees (hip and knee joints both).
Lift the upper torso, but keep the lower back flat on the ground. Try to lift
your chest toward the ceiling rather than forward. Hold for a second, then
slowly return to start. Repeat. This is not a large motion, and the lower
back should not lift off the ground.

E10   Static Crunch

Introduced WO#   26
Occurrences in program: 2
Primary muscle groups: Abdominals

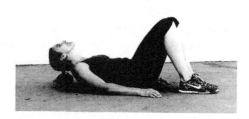

Almost identical to the regular Crunch: Lie down flat on your back, legs at
90 degrees (hip and knee joints both). Lift the upper torso, but keep the
lower back flat on the ground. Try to lift your chest toward the ceiling
rather than forward. Hold.

E11   Reverse Crunch

Introduced WO#   10
Occurrences in program: 3
Primary muscle groups: Abdominals

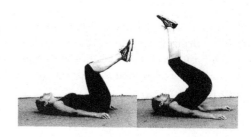

Lie down on your back and place your hands on the floor. Bring the knees
in towards the chest until they're bent to 90 degrees, with feet together.
Contract the abs to curl the hips off the floor. Lower and repeat. It's a
small movement, so try to use your abs to lift your hips rather than
swinging your legs for momentum.

E12   Unicycle Crunch

Introduced WO#	17
Occurrences in program:	13
Primary muscle groups:	Anterior chain

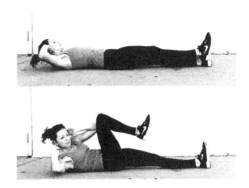

Here's the thing: A bicycle crunch is an abs exercise where you alternately bend one leg and stretch the other, while touching the bent knee with the opposite elbow. Now, if you only do that to one side repeatedly (e.g. right elbow to left knee), that would be a… Unicycle! Obviously you'd better alternate each set to keep things even.

E13   Bicycle Crunch

Introduced WO#	19
Occurrences in program:	2
Primary muscle groups:	Anterior chain

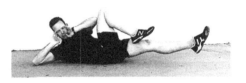

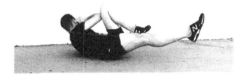

The Bicycle Crunch is an abs exercise where you alternately bend one leg and stretch the other, while touching the bent knee with the opposite elbow The lower back should not lift off the ground; focus on twisting more than lifting.

E14   Rower Sit-Up

Introduced WO#	1
Occurrences in program:	14
Primary muscle groups:	Anterior chain

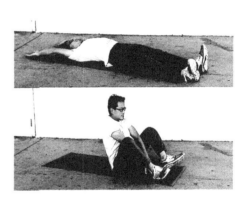

Rumor has it that the US Army has replaced the traditional Sit-Up with the Rower Sit-Up in its physical fitness tests. Lie on your back with arms extended overhead, legs straight and feet touching. In one motion, bring feet toward body while sitting up and swinging arms forward. In final position, extend arms and touch the ground between your feet with your fingertips. Return to start position; repeat sequence.

E15   Sit-Up

Introduced WO#	31
Occurrences in program:	6
Primary muscle groups:	Anterior chain

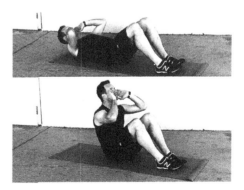

A classic. Probably not the best abs exercise, but worth a shot occasionally. Lie down flat on your back. Bend the knees to 90 degrees. Keep your hands loosely behind your ears. Sit up until your elbows are vertically aligned with your knees. Lie back down and repeat.

E16   Sit-Up Twist

Introduced WO#   34
Occurrences in program: 4
Primary muscle groups: Anterior chain; Obliques

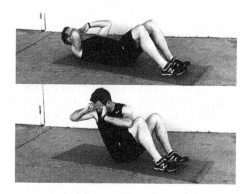

Also a classic. Performed almost in the same way as the Sit-Up, except you twist into the upper position so that one elbow ends up on the outside of the opposite knee. Lie back down and repeat, either to the same side for a unilateral motion, or to the other side for a bilateral motion.

E17   Russian Twist

Introduced WO#   22
Occurrences in program: 3
Primary muscle groups: Anterior chain; Obliques

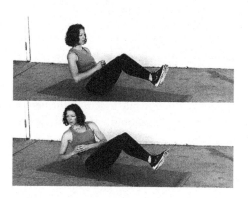

Sit on the floor with your knees bent and heels in light contact with or just off the ground. Lean back until you feel the abdominals engage to stabilize your body. Rotate as far as possible to one side and reach for the ground behind you. Make sure you rotate your entire torso and are not just reaching around with your arms. Change direction and move to the other side.

E18   KB Russian Twist

Introduced WO#   67
Occurrences in program: 8
Primary muscle groups: Anterior chain; Obliques

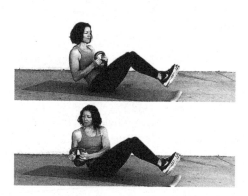

Start seated on the floor with your knees bent and heels in light contact with the ground. Lean back until you feel the abdominals engage to stabilize your body. Holding a medicine ball or kettlebell, rotate as far as possible to one side and reach toward the ground behind you. Make sure you rotate your entire torso and don't just reach around with your arms. Change direction and move the load to the other side. This exercise is more effective when performed slowly.

E19   Seated Leg Raise

Introduced WO#   11
Occurrences in program: 4
Primary muscle groups: Anterior chain

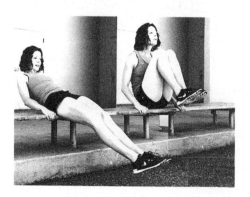

Leg Raises work the frontal hip and abdominal area (anterior chain) in a much more natural way than conventional sit-ups. Si ton the edge of a bench or chair. Lean back slightly and extend your leg down and forward. In a deliberate and controlled manner, lift your legs and pull the knees toward the chest. Return to start. Maintain perfect balance throughout.

E20   Flat Leg Raise

Introduced WO#	62
Occurrences in program:	6
Primary muscle groups:	Anterior chain

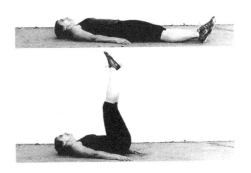

Leg Raises work the frontal hip and abdominal area (anterior chain) in a much more natural way than conventional sit-ups. The Flat Leg Raise is performed, as you might have deducted, from a position flat on your back. It is more challenging than the seated leg raise, but much less so than the Hanging Leg Raise. In a controlled manner, lift your straight legs until you get close to a perfect L-shape. This does require some flexibility; if your lower back starts rounding, don't go further, or flex your knees slightly.

E21   Hanging Leg Raise

Introduced WO#	68
Occurrences in program:	2
Primary muscle groups:	Anterior chain

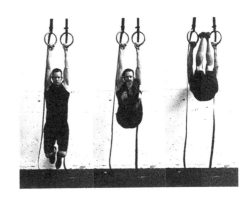

Hanging from a bar or gymnastic rings, lift your straight legs in a controlled manner until you get close to a perfect L-shape. This does require some flexibility. Don't move too fast. For an easier variety, bend your knees and tuck toward the chest. For a more challenging variety, lift your legs all the way up until your toes or ankles touch the bar.

E22   Inverted Ab Tuck

Introduced WO#	50
Occurrences in program:	6
Primary muscle groups:	Anterior chain

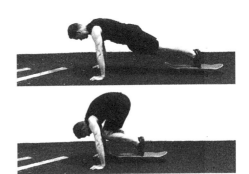

With your feet suspended on a swing or Pilates ball, or resting on a skateboard or similar, start from the upper push-up position. Use your abdominal muscles to pull your knees forward toward the chest, i.e. *tuck*. Try to rotate at the shoulder so your hips come up high, almost like you are about to do a handstand. Hold for a second, and then slowly return to start.

E23   Ab Roll-Out

Introduced WO#	88
Occurrences in program:	3
Primary muscle groups:	Anterior chain

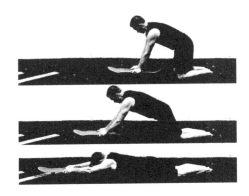

Kneel down and rest your hands on a moveable object. You can use a wheel, a barbell, TRX, gymnastic rings, a skateboard, or even playground swings. Push forward and stretch out as far forward as you can without letting your hips or torso touch the ground, then return to the starting position in a controlled manner. If you need more of a challenge, do it with only your toes touching the ground.

E24 KB Floor Wiper

Introduced WO#   59
Occurrences in program: 9
Primary muscle groups: Anterior chain

Start with a KB Floor Press as described (A13). Lock out the elbows in the upper press and maintain the position of the bells throughout. Keep your legs straight (1), lift them and simultaneously twist until your right shin gets close to the left kettlebell (2), then return to the ground (3). Repeat to the other side (4).

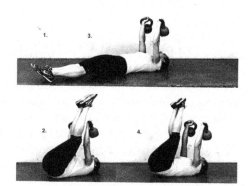

E25 KB Turkish Sit-Up

Introduced WO#   51
Occurrences in program: 6
Primary muscle groups: Anterior chain

The KB Turkish Sit-Up comprises the first and last three steps of the Turkish Get-Up: (1) Flat on your back, KB pressed to a straight arm, same knee bent, passive arm out. (2) Roll over onto the passive arm elbow. (3) Sit up, straightening the passive arm. Keep the KB arm vertical throughout, and do not move the foot of the bent leg. Do each step in reverse to return to the initial position.

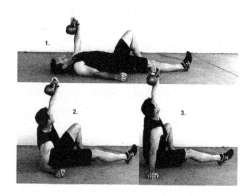

E26 KB Turkish Half-Up

Introduced WO#   85
Occurrences in program: 3
Primary muscle groups: Anterior chain; Posterior chain; Shoulders

The KB Turkish Half-Up comprises the first and last four steps of the Turkish Get-Up. (1) Flat on your back, KB pressed to a straight arm, same knee bent, passive arm out. (2) Roll over onto the passive arm elbow. (3) Sit up, straightening the passive arm. (4) Lift the hips to full extension. Keep the KB arm vertical throughout, and do not move the foot of the bent leg. Do each step in reverse to return to the initial position.

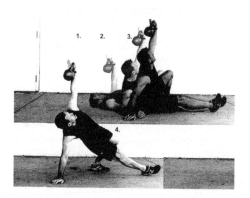

E27 KB Turkish Get-Up

Introduced WO#   109
Occurrences in program: 7
Primary muscle groups: Anterior chain; Posterior chain; Shoulders

The Turkish Get-Up starts with a Turkish Half-Up (steps 1-4). From (4) the hip lift position; (5) Pull the forward leg back under and put the knee to the ground; (6) Straighten up in a low lunge with the knee firmly on the ground; and (7) Stand up straight with the kettlebell overhead. From this position, retrace the steps in reverse until you are flat on your back.

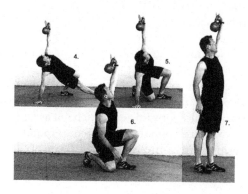

F. Posterior Chain Exercises

F01   Hurdles

Introduced WO#   33
Occurrences in program: 8
Primary muscle groups: Hips

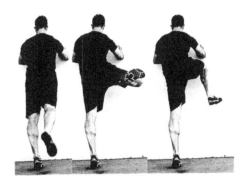

This is an excellent exercise for improving hip mobility, frequently used as a warm-up for track athletes.. Stand on the balls of your feet. Support yourself with your hands against a wall. Swing one leg straight back, and then pull the knee forward and high. When the knee is straight in front of the hip, extend the leg downward and back to the starting position. Try to achieve a smooth, fluid motion throughout. Switch sides and repeat.

F02   Dirty Dog

Introduced WO#   17
Occurrences in program: 8
Primary muscle groups: Glutes; Hips

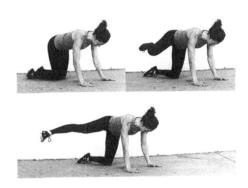

Get on your hands and knees. Tighten the midsection and lift one knee straight out to side. When you reach as high as you can without twisting the hip, extend the lower leg. Reverse and return to start, repeat on the other side.

F03   Down Dog / Up Dog

Introduced WO#   5
Occurrences in program: 19
Primary muscle groups: Hips; Core

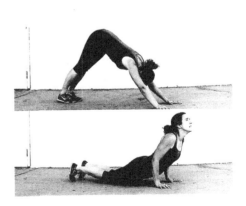

This is a dynamic version of two yoga staples, the Downward Facing Dog and the Upward Facing Dog. You start from the High Plank position (E01). Hinge at the hips and push them slowly up and back. Keep the lower back straight; you will likely feel a stretch along the backside of your legs. Hold for a second, then slowly come forward until the front of your hips are is close to the ground. Look up with the chest high, push the hips forward and hold for a second. Repeat.

F04   Bird Dog

Introduced WO#   17
Occurrences in program: 9
Primary muscle groups: Posterior chain

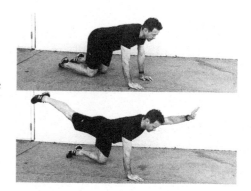

From a position on your hands and knees, stretch one leg and the opposite arm straight out. Keep the midsection tight throughout. Return to start, switch sides and repeat.

F05   Straight Bridge, Static

Introduced WO#   2
Occurrences in program: 7
Primary muscle groups: Posterior chain

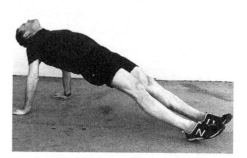

Start from a seated position with your legs straight out in front of you. Resting on your hands with straight arms, lift the hips as high as you can. Although you obviously could do this in a dynamic fashion too, i.e. lifting multiple times in a row, it is just as effective to just hold the upper position in a static lift, almost like a reverse Plank.

F06   Glute Bridge

Introduced WO#   1
Occurrences in program: 10
Primary muscle groups: Posterior chain

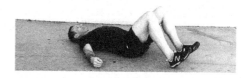

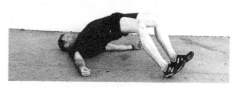

Glute Bridges use the shoulders as the foundation for the bridge lift and hence puts no load on the arms and hands. Push through the heels and lift the hips as high as you can; you should feel an intense contraction of the glutes. There are several ways to make this exercise more challenging: The simplest is to do them on one leg at a time. Elevating your leg(s) will make these more demanding.

F07   Elev. Glute Bridge

Introduced WO#   50
Occurrences in program: 3
Primary muscle groups: Posterior chain

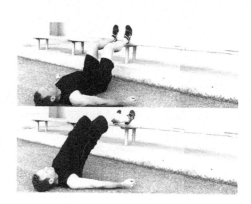

Elevating your leg(s) will make these more demanding than the conventional Glute Bridge (F06). Place your heels on a low bench or similar. Glute Bridges use the shoulders as the foundation for the bridge lift and hence puts no load on the arms and hands. Push through the heels and lift the hips as high as you can; you should feel an intense contraction of the glutes. You could do these on one leg at a time for a more challenging exercise.

F08   SL Glute Bridge

Introduced WO#   10
Occurrences in program: 7
Primary muscle groups: Posterior chain

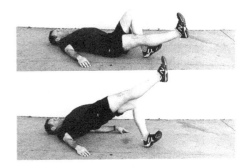

Nearly identical to the conventional Glute Bridge (F06), but using just one leg at the time to execute the lift makes the Single Leg Glute Bridge considerably more challenging. Stretch one leg out straight and bend the other to approximately 90 degrees. Push through the heel and lift the hips as high as you can. Switch and repeat on the next rep or set.

F09   Band Deadlift

Introduced WO#   47
Occurrences in program: 3
Primary muscle groups: Posterior chain

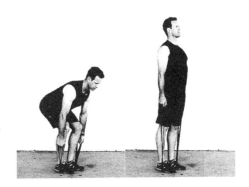

Place a rubber resistance band on the ground and step onto it with both feet, shoulder width apart. Leave an equal loop of the band on each side and bend over to grab the ends with your hands. Straighten your back and brace your midsection. Stand up, keeping the lower back straight and your midsection tight throughout. Reverse and repeat.

F10   KB Sumo Deadlift

Introduced WO#   67
Occurrences in program: 3
Primary muscle groups: Posterior chain; Legs

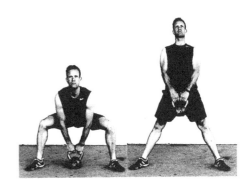

Deadlifts represent a fundamental skill: Lifting something heavy from the ground to hip height. The Sumo stance is wide, with the feet pointing out about 45 degrees. Grab a heavy kettlebell, straighten your back and brace your midsection. Stand up, keeping the lower back straight and your midsection tight throughout. Reverse and repeat. Keep your chest and chin up.

F11   KB Deadlift

Introduced WO#   50
Occurrences in program: 19
Primary muscle groups: Posterior chain; Legs; Shoulders

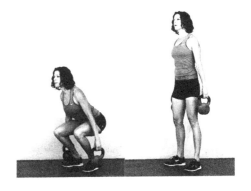

Maintain a tight midsection with the back straight, shoulders low and back, and the chest held high. The conventional KB Deadlift requires two kettlebells. Stand with your feet shoulder-width apart and the KBs just outside of the forefoot on each side. Straighten your back and brace your midsection. Stand up, keeping the lower back straight and your midsection tight throughout. Reverse and repeat. Keep your chest and chin up.

F12   KB SL Deadlift

Introduced WO#   26
Occurrences in program: 11
Primary muscle groups: Posterior chain; Legs (hamstrings)

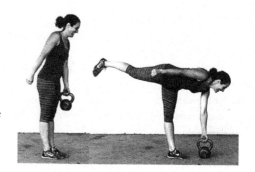

The KB SL Deadlift is a variety of straight leg deadlifts, and a superb exercise for training balance and hamstring strength. Stand up with a kettlebell held straight down in one hand. Shift your weight to the side holding the bell, then hinge forward until the bell touches the ground. The arm should remain vertical, whereas the unloaded leg is kept straight and aligned with the torso.

F13   KB 2h Swing

Introduced WO#   11
Occurrences in program: 24
Primary muscle groups: Posterior chain; Core; Lower arms

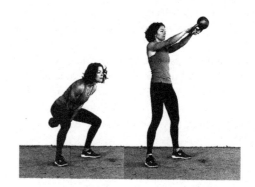

The foundation for all kettlebell work; helps develop strong posterior chain muscles. The stance is slightly wider than shoulder width. Hold the bell with both hands, dip down in the knees, and swing the bell back between your legs. Quickly straighten up and drive the hips forward, but don't lean back. You don't actively lift the bell, all the force comes from the hips and the arms function as a lever. Swing up to about the height of your forehead, and keep your midsection tight throughout.

F14   KB 1h Swing

Introduced WO#   17
Occurrences in program: 17
Primary muscle groups: Posterior chain; Core; Lower arms

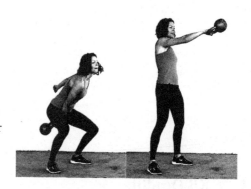

Performed just like the 2-handed KB Swing, but using just one hand. Remember that you should not lean forward; focus instead on sticking your butt out. All the force comes from the hips, you don't actively lift the bell with the arm. Keep the passive arm to the side; avoid resting it on your thigh.

F15   KB H2H Swing

Introduced WO#   70
Occurrences in program: 8
Primary muscle groups: Posterior chain; Core; Lower arms

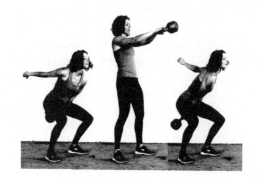

The H2H (hand-to-hand) swing starts like a single-handed kettlebell swing. As the bell slows its ascent and reaches its apex, you reach forward and switch to the other hand. The motion should be quick and efficient, almost like a karate punch.

F16   KB High Swing

Introduced WO#   48
Occurrences in program: 8
Primary muscle groups: Posterior chain; Core; Lower arms

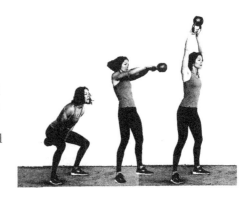

The High Kettlebell Swing is sometimes referred to as American Kettlebell Swing. Compared to the conventional 2-handed swing (F13), this requires a more forceful thrust to swing the bell higher. However, it is also not quite as fast. Do a kettlebell swing as described above, but swing the bell all the way up overhead. Be careful not to let the bell move too far back, as you may lose stability and injure your shoulders.

F17   KB Clean

Introduced WO#   17
Occurrences in program: 21
Primary muscle groups: Posterior chain; Core

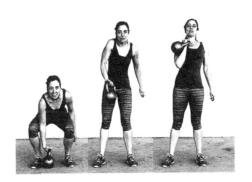

Another fundamental exercise that must be mastered before moving onto more advanced kettlebell exercises. This lift starts with the bell on the ground. Grab the handle with one hand and tighten your core. Pull the bell quickly up into the rack position, i.e. upper arm firmly against your torso and thumb knuckle against the collarbone. The bell should rest against your outer forearm and biceps, with the arm firmly bent. Return the bell to the ground in a controlled motion for a dead clean (preferred), or swing between your legs for continuous swing cleans.

F18   KB Clean & Press

Introduced WO#   23
Occurrences in program: 23
Primary muscle groups: Posterior chain; Core; Shoulders;
                                Arms

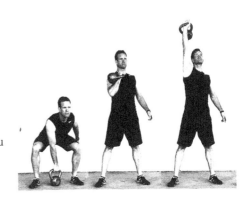

Simply put: You're combining the KB Clean (F17) with the KB Press (A14). Perform a clean to the rack position as described above. With your core muscles tight, press the bell overhead in a controlled motion until you lock out the elbow. Keep your core tight. Return the bell to the rack position, then back to the ground. Repeat.

F19　Windmill

Introduced WO#　　　　　　　47
Occurrences in program:　　4
Primary muscle groups:　　Posterior chain; Obliques

Stand with a wide stance and the arms straight out to the sides at shoulder height. Push the hips back (hinge) whilst twisting the torso. Try to maintain the arm position and keep pushing the hips back until you can touch the ground. Reverse and repeat on the opposite side.

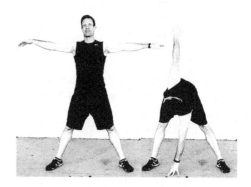

F20　KB Low Windmill

Introduced WO#　　　　　　　96
Occurrences in program:　　3
Primary muscle groups:　　Posterior chain; Obliques

KB Windmill as described below (F21), except you hold the kettlebell in the lower hand. This is considerably easier but you sacrifice the stabilizing training for the shoulder joint. The Low Windmill is a good exercise to work on if you have challenges with hip or hamstring flexibility, or shoulder stability; when this is sorted out you can go on to the conventional KB Windmill, using a lightweight kettlebell at first.

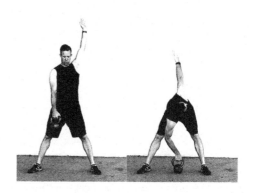

F21　KB Windmill

Introduced WO#　　　　　　　68
Occurrences in program:　　5
Primary muscle groups:　　Posterior chain; Shoulders; Obliques

"The windmill should be a simultaneous hip hinging and spine rotation", according to Pavel Tsatsouline, the father of modern US kettlebell training. You start with the bell pressed overhead and the elbow locked out. Stand with a wide stance; push the hips back whilst twisting the torso to maintain the vertical arm. Come down as far as you can without bending your back, legs, or losing control of the arm. It helps to keep your eyes on the kettlebell at all times. Reverse and stand back up in a controlled manner. Go light at first; substitute with F20 if needed.

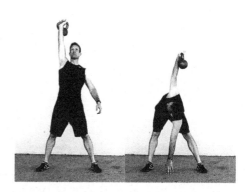

F22　Sledgehammer

Introduced WO#　　　　　　　97
Occurrences in program:　　2
Primary muscle groups:　　Posterior chain; Anterior chain;
　　　　　　　　　　　　　　Shoulders

You got it – just like Granddad used to do. Most people have a preference, for instance the right hand closest to the sledgehammer head and the left foot forward: Make sure you also switch and do it the other way around for the same amount of reps. It is beneficial to have something to hit, say an old car tire. Unless you really want to smash something, obviously. Try to make the motion fluid, fast and powerful.

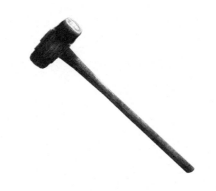

G. Complex Motion Exercises

G01   Model Walk

Introduced WO#   34
Occurrences in program: 7
Primary muscle groups:

Imagine that you are wearing 4-inch heels and must prove to the highway patrol officer that, despite appearances, you are certainly not intoxicated on too many vodka martinis and can walk in a perfectly straight line with impeccable grace and a haughtily raised chin. Keep the chest high and shoulders low and back. The hardest part is keeping a straight face.

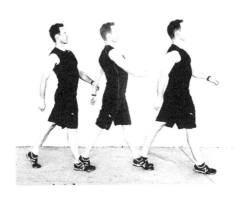

G02   Chaplin Walk

Introduced WO#   34
Occurrences in program: 7
Primary muscle groups:

Feet and knees turned out as far as you can, Charlie Chaplin-style. The speed should be like a 1920ies film reel. Stay on the balls of your feet. Hilarious mustache is optional.

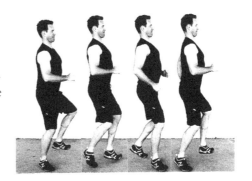

G03   Rooster Walk

Introduced WO#   52
Occurrences in program: 5
Primary muscle groups:

A hankering for the Kremlin, anyone? On the balls of your feet, walk with straight legs, kicking up to about hip height. Be careful not to overextend as you could easily tear a hamstring muscle if they're tight.

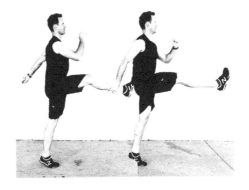

G04   Crab Walk

Introduced WO#   34
Occurrences in program: 7
Primary muscle groups:

On your hands and feet with your back to the ground. Lift the hips and move forward or backward. Strictly speaking, of course, a crab walks sideways – but let's not get too pedantic about this.

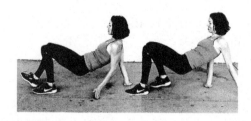

G05   Bear Walk

Introduced WO#   4
Occurrences in program: 8
Primary muscle groups:

Crawl forward on your hands and feet. Knees should not touch the ground; keep your hips high.

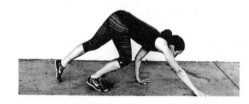

G06   Wheelbarrow

Introduced WO#   34
Occurrences in program: 10
Primary muscle groups:

Back to the playground: Start from the high plank position. Have a friend grab your ankles. Walk forward on your hands. Keep your midsection tight and the body straight at all times; try not to slouch, twist, or stick your butt up.

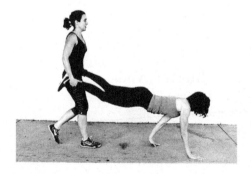

G07   KB Farmer Walk

Introduced WO#   70
Occurrences in program: 6
Primary muscle groups:

This is as simple as it gets: Just hold a kettlebell in each hand and take them for a walk. Keep your arms straight down. That's pretty much it. However, you need to pay attention to your shoulders: Stick your chest out, with the shoulders back and low and the chin held high. Think Pamela Anderson in Baywatch, and you get the general idea.

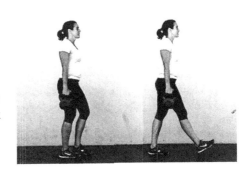

G08   KB Rack Walk

Introduced WO#   70
Occurrences in program: 2
Primary muscle groups:

Clean the kettlebell(s) to the rack position, i.e. cradled against the upper arm. Walk.

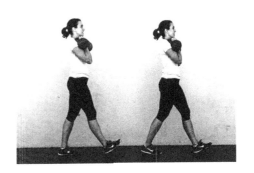

G09   KB Waiter Walk

Introduced WO#   70
Occurrences in program: 3
Primary muscle groups:

The Waiter Walk is pretty straightforward. Press one or two kettlebell(s) overhead. Lock out the elbow. Walk, maintaining a tight midsection and straight arms at all times.

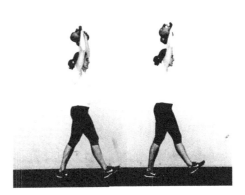

G10 KB Pick-Up Walk

Introduced WO#   61
Occurrences in program: 3
Primary muscle groups:

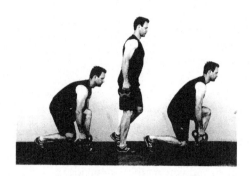

Hold a bell in each hand with your arms down along your side. Take a normal step forward and touch ground with the bells, crouching with split legs (but don't do a lunge). Hold on to the bells and straighten up as you take another step forward with the opposite leg. Touch ground with the bells, straighten and take another step, etc etc. Obviously, this can also be done with a single kettlebell.

G11 Buddy Carry

Introduced WO#   65
Occurrences in program: 5
Primary muscle groups:

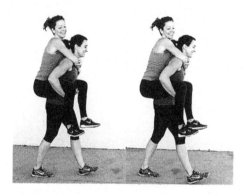

Have your workout buddy hop onto your back and hold on tight. Walk. It is generally best if you have reasonably similar body weights.

G12 Buddy Pull

Introduced WO#   59
Occurrences in program: 10
Primary muscle groups:

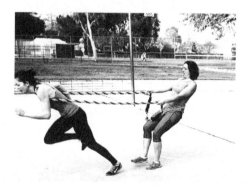

Wrap a thick rope across your shoulders and have your workout buddy hold onto the ends and provide some resistance. The person holding the reins is responsible for making the exercise flow, i.e. don't hold back too hard. Run on the balls of your feet, keeping the step frequency high. It should be a sprint more than a grind. If you're on your own, tying some kettlebells to your towing rope works great. Or you could load up an old snow sled with kettlebells or rocks.

G13 Reverse Buddy Pull

Introduced WO#   87
Occurrences in program: 6
Primary muscle groups:

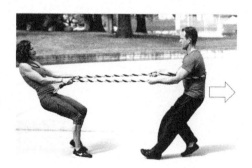

Loop the rope around your waist and let your workout buddy hold the ends. Bend your knees to lower your hips a little and walk backwards. This is a slower motion than the sprinting action of the conventional Buddy Pull, and will be an equally good workout for your friend trying to hold you back.

G14   Run-In-Place (R.I.P.)

Introduced WO#   4
Occurrences in program: 4
Primary muscle groups:

It is exactly what it sounds like: You run. In one place, i.e. without moving forward. Keep your posture upright, stay on the balls of your feet, and lift your knees moderately high. Don't crouch. Focus on keeping the frequency up.

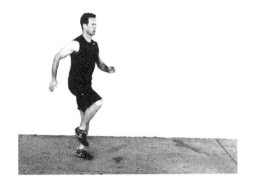

G15   Run

Introduced WO#   22
Occurrences in program: 13
Primary muscle groups:

It is up to you, but we typically mean "run really fast", i.e. sprint. Remember: Sprinting happens on the balls of your feet and the heels should not touch ground but briefly. You should definitely not land on your heels! Execution is fast and powerful with knees driven high.

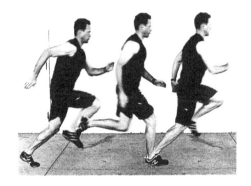

G16   Medicine Ball Toss

Introduced WO#   58
Occurrences in program: 5
Primary muscle groups:

Grab a medicine ball. Toss it. Try to find a number of different ways to throw it. For efficiency it is best if you pair up with someone and throw the ball to each other. Alternatively, run after the ball to pick it back up. Medicine balls come in a variety of makes and weights. A large, padded ball with a weight of 5-10 kg (10-20 lbs) is good for throwing. The Medicine Ball Toss can work well as a general warm-up.

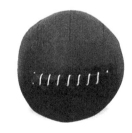

ABOUT THE AUTHOR

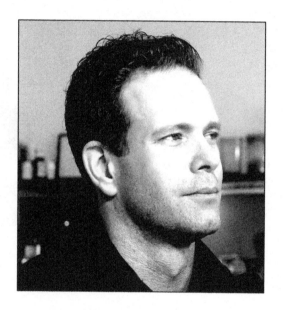

Alf Berle is the founder and head coach of the Nordic Method workout system. Growing up in the majestic fjord landscape of western Norway, Alf was a competitive athlete and coach well into his twenties. After suffering the debilitating consequences of a sedentary decade as an office worker he decided to put his coaching skills back in use, with himself as the primary guinea pig. Several years were spent researching and testing various training schemes, and he eventually designed a program that would restore functional fitness and be sustainable for decades. As a community-based fitness initiative, the Nordic Method was founded in Palo Alto, CA, in 2013. Workout groups are now established there and in several European locations. Alf is a certified training instructor by the Norwegian Confederation of Sports and a certified athletics coach by the Norwegian Athletics Association.